The
Student Nurse
Toolkit

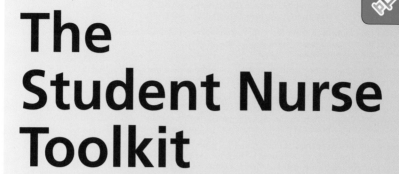

The Student Nurse Toolkit

AN ESSENTIAL GUIDE FOR SURVIVING YOUR COURSE

Professor Ian Peate

EN(G), RGN, DipN(Lond), RNT, BE (Hons), MA(Lond), LLM
Editor-in-Chief, *British Journal of Nursing*
Visiting Professor, University of West London

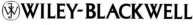
WILEY-BLACKWELL
A John Wiley & Sons, Ltd., Publication

This edition first published 2013
© 2013 by John Wiley & Sons, Ltd

Registered office: John Wiley & Sons, Ltd, The Atrium, Southern Gate, Chichester, West
                       Sussex, PO19 8SQ, UK

Editorial offices: 9600 Garsington Road, Oxford, OX4 2DQ, UK
                       The Atrium, Southern Gate, Chichester, West Sussex, PO19 8SQ, UK
                       111 River Street, Hoboken, NJ 07030-5774, USA

For details of our global editorial offices, for customer services and for information about how
to apply for permission to reuse the copyright material in this book please see our website at
www.wiley.com/wiley-blackwell

Library of Congress Cataloging-in-Publication Data
Peate, Ian.
  The student nurse toolkit : an essential guide for surviving your course / Ian Peate.
     p. ; cm.
  Includes bibliographical references and index.
  ISBN 978-1-118-39378-9 (softback : alk. paper)—ISBN 978-1-118-39389-5—
ISBN 978-1-118- 39390-1 (Mobi)—ISBN 978-1-118-39391-8 (PDF)—
ISBN 978-1-118-39392-5 (Pub)—ISBN 978-1-118-69030-7
  I. Title.
  [DNLM: 1. Education, Nursing—methods. 2. Students, Nursing. 3. Vocational Guidance.WY 18]
  RT71
  610.73071—dc23
                                                                            2013013056

A catalogue record for this book is available from the British Library.

Wiley also publishes its books in a variety of electronic formats. Some content that appears in
print may not be available in electronic books.

Cover image: courtesy of Anthony Peate
Cover design by Sarah Dickinson

Set in Frutiger Roman 8.5/12pt by Aptara Inc., New Delhi, India
Printed in Singapore by Ho Printing Singapore Pte Ltd

1   2013

Contents

Dedication, vi

Acknowledgements, vi

Preface, vii

CHAPTER 1 Entry to Nursing, 1

CHAPTER 2 The Nursing and Midwifery Council and Other
Regulatory Bodies, 15

CHAPTER 3 Nursing Education: the Standards for Pre-registration
Nurse Education, 27

CHAPTER 4 Nursing, Health and Social Care, 43

CHAPTER 5 Assessment Tools, 60

CHAPTER 6 The Essential Skills Clusters, 79

CHAPTER 7 The University Setting, 98

CHAPTER 8 Practice Learning Opportunities, 115

CHAPTER 9 The Nursing Elective, 131

CHAPTER 10 Managing Self, 143

CHAPTER 11 Terminology: Terms Used in Healthcare, 162

CHAPTER 12 Evidence-Based Practice, 178

CHAPTER 13 Reflective Practice, 195

CHAPTER 14 Your Professional Portfolio, 212

CHAPTER 15 Records and Record Keeping, 230

CHAPTER 16 Protocols, Policies and Legal Matters, 249

CHAPTER 17 Clinical Academic Careers, 268

CHAPTER 18 Preceptorship and Continuing Professional Development, 281

CHAPTER 19 What Do I Do If...? Questions You Did Not Want To Ask
Out Loud, 298

Index, 313

Dedication

This text is dedicated to the cohort of student nurses known as September 1997 who studied at the University of Hertfordshire and have now moved onto great things.

Acknowledgements

To my partner Jussi Lahtinen who puts up with me. My dear friend Frances Cohen who continues to support all of my endeavours. My brother Anthony Peate who produced all of the illustrations for this text. The staff at the Royal College of Nursing Library London.

Preface

This book has been written for those who are considering nursing as a profession and those who are on a programme of study. This includes students at all stages of their programme. There may be some of you reading this who are about to go into their first staff nurse job, in which case congratulations Staff Nurse. Some readers may be going to university for the first time and some may be going into the clinical area as a novice nurse excited and anxious: both at the same time (yuk!).

In this little book I hope you will be able to find some of the answers to your questions, some reassurance about issues you might be facing on your course. The book will not provide answers to all of the challenges you face (I am only human) and anyway, I believe you have it in you to seek the solutions to the challenges you encounter: you just need to be prodded sometimes. I have been so lucky in my nursing career. It's the best job in the world (the pay isn't so good, though). I was lucky with the people I have been privileged to care for and to study with.

I am totally committed to you, the student, to teaching and learning from and with you and I am also committed to having a good laugh. I am devoted to the students I have been truly delighted to help learn the art and science of nursing, this thing (nursing) that defies definition, this thing that once it is in your blood is impossible to get rid of (I have warned you).

In these pages you will find some features that have been planned to help break up the blocks of text, to bring the pages alive and speak to you. Throughout the book there are the voices of many people: students and registered nurses who have shared their experiences with me (some of them were my role models). Like a good nurse I have ensured that confidentiality has been respected (I could give you a reference for this but, I won't). I have included pearls of wisdom (not all mine) that are intended to drop a hint here and there to help get you through. Dotted throughout are student activities. It is not essential you complete them, but you may find them helpful (don't worry, you won't be assessed on them!). Most of the various sections all have their own section summaries; I have done this so that you can recall quickly what has just been said. At the end of each chapter is a list of resources, websites that I have used in the past and which I hope you will also find useful. The most important resources, however, are the human resources all around you: your peers, the staff nurse who becomes your mentor, your preceptor, your lecturer, the patient and your family. Make the most of these precious resources, try not to abuse them. They are nuggets of gold and should be cherished.

I use the various terms patient, service user and client interchangeably throughout the text. I know this comes across as 'messy' but nursing can sometimes be like that, as can the people we care for, the most important thing (I think) is to remember that patients, clients, service users – whatever the term used – are people and they deserve the best and safest standards of care we can muster.

I hope this book provides a voice and context to the nursing experience in a way that is an easy read as well as an inspiration to you. I hope that you enjoy your nursing, the best job in the world….

You know you are a nurse when you watch *Casualty* or *Holby City* and to the annoyance of your family you point out all the mistakes that they have made!

You know you are a nurse when you are in Chapel Market shopping and a patient shouts across the street 'that's my nurse, he saved my life'.

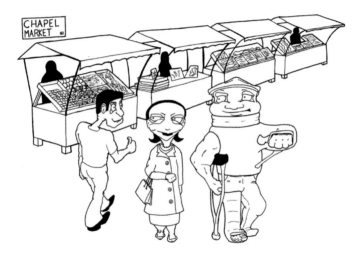

Ian Peate

London, March 2013

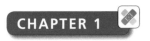

CHAPTER 1

 # Entry to Nursing

WHAT THIS CHAPTER CONTAINS

- An overview of the general entry requirements for pre-registration nurse education
- Pointers on helping you choose the right university
- Funding issues
- The selection process

> After all these years if you asked me to do it all again I would. Nursing is the best job I have ever done. *A recently retired registered nurse with over 40 years' nursing service*

This chapter starts with a comment from a nurse who has just retired after a 40-year nursing career, and it is shown as a means to inspire you when you are thinking of choosing nursing as your future career. You must also be aware, however, that nursing is not for everyone and that things have changed since this nurse started her training (it is no longer a training programme, but an educational process). Many people, both inside and outside of the profession, might say the changes have been for the better; some would suggest that they have been for the worse.

Nursing is a varied, challenging and rewarding career for those who would like to make a difference to the lives of people locally, nationally and internationally. Nurses and nursing staff take responsibility for the care they provide and answer for their own judgements and actions. They constantly respond to new challenges and act as a leader, carer and clinician.

Experienced nurses find fulfilling careers in positions of responsibility, often running nurse-led clinics or taking leadership roles up to executive level. Nursing is changing rapidly, with increasing focus on public health and disease prevention. It is possible to develop career pathways in clinical, research, education and management roles.

Nurses don't just work in hospitals. There are opportunities to work in, among others, GP surgeries, clinics, nursing and residential homes, occupational health

The Student Nurse Toolkit: An Essential Guide for Surviving Your Course, First Edition. Ian Peate.
© 2013 John Wiley & Sons, Ltd. Published 2013 by John Wiley & Sons, Ltd.

services, voluntary organisations that run hospices or residential care, and the pharmaceutical industry. Nurses also work in university education, on leisure cruise ships and in the military.

Some readers of this book will have embarked on a programme of nurse education already; this chapter aims to entice those who are thinking of nursing as a profession and provides information concerning the requirements needed to enrol successfully on a programme of study. For some this might seem like having to jump through hoops; however, knowing what hoops have to be jumped through is important!

There are over 90 universities (approved educational institutions) in the UK offering programmes of study that lead to registration. It takes 3 years to become a nurse unless a student is able to demonstrate that they have already met some of the course requirements (sometimes called advanced standing). Nurse education is based in the universities and is delivered in direct partnership with NHS Trusts and other organisations (for example, the independent and voluntary sector), which provides nursing students with practice learning opportunities in health and social care settings.

The education programme is split 50/50: 50% is spent in practice, so that students are able to learn how to provide direct nursing care. The remaining 50% of the programme is spent learning the knowledge and technical abilities needed to underpin and support practice, usually on a university campus.

There are four fields of nursing and you need to decide upon the field in which you intend to register:

- ☧ learning disabilities,
- ☧ mental health,
- ☧ children,
- ☧ adult.

SECTION SUMMARY

There are four fields of nursing. All nursing programmes are offered to degree level. Nursing is practised where ever there are people, so the notion of nursing being solely hospital-based is outdated.

 ## Your university of choice

Choosing the right university for your nursing studies will depend on a number of factors. Below is a list of what you may need to consider or take into account.

- ☧ Does the university offer the field in which I intend to register?
- ☧ Is the geographical location suitable?
- ☧ What placement opportunities are on offer?

- 🜪 Do I have the right entry requirements? (i.e. UCAS points.)
- 🜪 Does it have good quality assurance processes? (Include the university's reputation.)
- 🜪 What does the Nursing and Midwifery Council (NMC) say about the university? (Go and look at their website.)
- 🜪 What do the various quality assurance bodies say about the university? (For example, the Quality Assurance Agency.)

Remember that your choice of university can be a life-changing decision, so do as much research as you can: choose the right course and the right university for the right reason.

> I went to six university open days before settling on the university I am at now; the thing that clinched it for me here was that they provide excellent practice learning opportunities. I go out working with the homeless sometimes and working with vulnerable families, it's a great opportunity. *Second year mental health nursing student*

Take time making you decision, think about where you will be happy. Do you want to be close to home or are you looking to live in a different part of the country? Be sure, however, that you do not take too much time pondering your choice: there are specific deadlines that must be met to ensure entry for the next academic year.

> I had no choice really with my university. I have two young kids, so it was the local university for me. *First year mental health nursing student*

SECTION SUMMARY

Be sure to do your homework and to check out the universities to which you are thinking of applying. Do they offer what you want? Consider carefully the field of nursing that you are going to apply for and, most importantly, the reasons for your choice.

Funding

Current funding arrangements to undertake a BSc Nursing degree vary in the four countries of the UK. Since September 2012 English and Welsh funding arrangements have been to provide a non-means-tested grant and a means-tested bursary to new students.

Nursing students can access additional support in the form of a maintenance loan. In addition, students can apply for a number of extra allowances if they meet specific criteria. These allowances include support for disabled students and for those with dependent adults and children. The NHS will continue to pay all course fees. There are, however, certain requirements to qualify for this financial assistance. Applicants must:

- have been resident in the UK throughout the 3 years preceding the first day of the academic year of the course, other than for the purpose of receiving full-time education,
- have settled status in the UK within the meaning of the UK Immigration Act 1971, on the first academic year of the course,
- be ordinarily resident in the UK on the first day of the first academic year of the course.

Similar arrangements are in place for students studying in Scotland and Northern Ireland. You should check the appropriate websites and speak to the university of your choice for up-to-date information concerning fees and funding.

Meeting requirements

Once you have chosen a university you need to be accepted onto the course. There are a number of requirements that you must meet, some of which will be prescribed by the university and others by the NMC.

The NMC leave the entry requirements to each university. There are no national minimum academic entry requirements for entry into nursing programmes; each university sets its own criteria. All applicants have to be able to demonstrate evidence of literacy and numeracy.

For numeracy this includes evidence of the ability to accurately manipulate numbers as applied to volume, weight and length (including addition, subtraction, division and multiplication, and use of decimals, fractions and percentages). For literacy you must provide evidence of the ability to read and comprehend English (or Welsh, as applicable) and to communicate clearly and effectively in writing, including using a word processor. If you have a disability then the above can be met through the use of reasonable adjustments.

It is important that you check with each university prior to applying to see whether your qualifications meet its entry criteria. As a general guide, most universities are looking for the following qualifications or their equivalent: you will usually need a minimum of five GCSEs at grade C or above (usually this includes English language or literature and a science subject), plus two A levels or their equivalent (in reality you may need three A levels, so you must check with the university directly).

Having satisfied yourself (and ultimately the university) that you meet the minimum criteria you need to submit your application form. Universities receive thousands of applications from able candidates wishing to undertake nursing programmes, but they all have a specific target number of students to recruit. Your application needs to stand out from the crowd and make an impact so that it is put on the invite-to-interview pile rather than the rejected pile.

The application form

The application form is the only thing your prospective university will have to judge you on, so it is important to take your time over this aspect of the application (remember that the application form is only one part of the whole process). The form will have several pages and some of the questions may seem daunting. Admissions tutors (the people who make the initial decision to proceed or not with your application) receive thousands of applications to sift through: yours has to catch their eye. Application forms are designed to give you an opportunity to sell yourself and you should keep this in mind at all times when deciding how to answer the questions posed.

> I spend 4 to 6 hours a day looking at application forms and I can spot a good one a mile off and a bad one five miles off.
> *Admissions tutor, BSc(Hons) Nursing*

1 First do your research about the university, the programme, the profession and the practice learning opportunities.
2 When registering online remember your username and answers to any security questions; for example, passwords.
3 Be sure to read all aspects of the application and any instructions provided.
4 When you are asked to make your choices, think carefully: choose the correct institution and the correct course.
5 Include all of your employment and educational details; if there are any gaps be prepared to account for them.
6 The personal statement, it could be suggested, is the most important aspect of the form. Do not type your statement straight into this section: write it first with a word processor or similar, using the spell-check facility, and copy and paste it into the form when you are ready. Use Times New Roman, font size 12.
7 Be concise, do not waffle and be sure that it is all your own work. Plagiarism is easily detected using specialised software.
8 When you think it is finished, click Preview to see what it will look like when an admissions tutor sees it. Edit it if you want to make any changes.
9 Ensure your application is submitted before the set deadline.
10 Fill in all parts of the form: if any sections are not relevant to you then write 'not applicable'.
11 Proofread the form carefully before you submit it: pressing the Send button has the ability to change the rest of your life.
12 Make sure that your e-mail address is appropriate: remember the admissions tutor and others will see it, so do not use anything crude or rude.

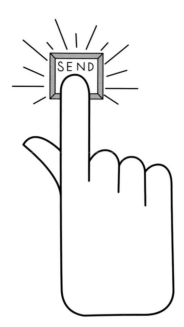

Here are 10 things not to put on your CV.
1 You pet's name
2 Your favourite colour
3 Somebody else's details (copy and pasting)
4 Hobbies: getting drunk and singing karaoke
5 The fact that you once won a strawberry-eating contest
6 The ability to say the alphabet backwards in under 4 seconds
7 I am a perfectionist and rarely, if ever, forget details
8 Languages: speak fluent English and Spinach
9 Reason for leaving my last job: pushed out so the new boss could give the job to her boyfriend.
10 References: please do not contact my immediate line manager at my current job. My colleagues will provide me with a better reference.

Selection day

Well done, you have been successful at getting an interview, but there are still a number of other hoops through which you must jump. The best piece of advice for you at this stage is to *be prepared*. You have to do your homework. Usual guidance would include:

- know where the interview is being held (the address and building),
- know where the interview will take place (the room in the building),
- be on time,
- dress appropriately (no jeans or trainers): be smart and professional,
- avoid multiple earrings, nose rings, or lip and tongue piercings,
- bring the appropriate original documentation (not photocopies).

Nursing selection days require more of candidates than conventional interviews. Selection days are run differently at different universities; some may require you to do some preliminary work, maybe online, prior to the face-to-face meeting. The aim of the selection day is to ensure that you are suitable for the programme of study, that you understand that you are about to commit yourself to 3 years' hard work and that you can manage the demands of the programme. You must be able to communicate with the selection panel that you know that nursing is not what you see on *Holby City* or *ER*. The selection day is also your opportunity to see whether the university is good enough for you. This means you have to have attitude, *good attitude*. Having done your homework you will have discovered:

- the fields of nursing offered,
- the timetable for the selection day (they usually last at least 4 to 6 hours),
- the documentation you have been asked to bring with you,
- the methods of selection being used, such as aptitude test(s) (these may include psychometric testing), group interview and face-to-face interview,
- the placement opportunities available,
- information about the university.

All universities are required to ensure that applicants to pre-registration nursing programmes are of good health and good character sufficient for safe and effective practice as a nurse. You will be required to undergo a criminal records check; some universities do this before the programme commences and some do it when you have accepted a place on the programme. The check is carried out by the Criminal Records Bureau (or its equivalent) and you must confirm on your application that you agree to this being done; the provisions covered by the Rehabilitation of Offenders Act 1974 do not apply.

If you have a criminal conviction or a police caution you will not be barred automatically from securing a place on the programme and ultimately working in the NHS, as each conviction is considered in the light of all relevant circumstances. However, you must make known any criminal convictions or police cautions. You are usually asked to provide personal references vouching for your good character.

All applicants are subject to satisfactory health clearance prior to commencing any clinical placements. If you have a particular problem that you think may affect your ability to work or study, or if you have any questions about health requirements, you should contact the university to which you plan to apply.

The interview

Again, different universities use different techniques to interview and select their potential students. It is usual for a marking system of some sort to be used so that those interviewing (the panel) can make an objective decision concerning selection. You might be asked to take part in group interviews, individual interviews, or both.

Group interviews

Often four to six candidates are asked to discuss a topic, for example 'people with HIV should be isolated when being nursed'. Your discussion, as a group and as an individual, will be monitored by the interviewers, who could be university staff, clinical staff and service users. The purpose is to observe how you interact with others, how you listen and communicate verbally and, importantly, non-verbally, as well as what your opinions are and how you express them. The technique is to ensure that you are confident but not cocky, that you are articulate but respectful of others and that you have the capacity to work as a member of a team. Nurses are often asked to act as someone's advocate. To do this effectively – acting in a person's best interests – you have to be able to speak up for them. Remember this when you are being interviewed.

Individual interviews

These interviews will challenge your perception of nursing. The panel, made up of academics, clinicians and service users, will ask you questions designed to elicit your knowledge and insight, your ability to be caring and compassionate and your commitment to the proposed programme of study.

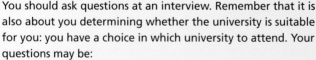
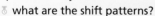
PEARLS OF WISDOM

You should ask questions at an interview. Remember that it is also about you determining whether the university is suitable for you: you have a choice in which university to attend. Your questions may be:
- what are the shift patterns?
- how much time is spent in the community setting versus the hospital setting?

- what are the bursary payments?
- please tell me about the assessment strategies used,
- what key areas of research are the department involved in?
- what support systems are in place for students?
- if appropriate, ask about student accommodation.

The only way to succeed at interview is to prepare. Do your homework. Ask questions. Be yourself. Do not undersell yourself. The panel want to get to know you: they already like you otherwise they would not have asked you to interview. Make it really clear why you want to study nursing. Be confident and demonstrate that you are the type of person who has the ability and the skills to make a positive difference to the lives of the people you will be caring for and the communities in which they live.

There are no trick questions at interview; the panel know and will expect you to be nervous. There are, however, questions that will test you. You will certainly be asked why you have chosen nursing and the specific field of nursing you have applied for.

PEARLS OF WISDOM

It would be unwise to respond to this question by saying you have always admired the nurses on *Casualty* or *Holby City*, or that you like the uniform.

Other questions may include:

- what do you think is the role of a nurse?
- what are the qualities of a good nurse?
- of those qualities, what is the most important quality in a nurse?
- where do you think nursing takes place? (Remember, it is wherever people are, not just in hospitals.)
- what is it you intend to get out of your studies at this university?
- what made you choose this university?
- what skills do you have that may make you suitable for this course?
- what experience of health and social care have you had?
- what are your strengths and weaknesses?
- how do you intend managing your time; what are your time-management skills like?
- how do you cope with stress?
- how do you handle criticism and cope with authority?

The panel may refer back to your performance at group interview; you may even be asked to elaborate on comments you made there, so be ready to do this. Remember that there are no trick questions: they are genuinely interested in your responses and how you present yourself. Be ready to convince the panel that you have the personal attributes that will help you make a success of the programme. Let them know how you are prepared to cope with the physical and intellectual demands such a programme requires, but remember to be realistic in your responses: do not make things up, and be honest. If during any stage of the interview you are unsure of the question being asked, then request that the question be repeated.

ACTIVITY 1.1

What is wrong with this question: 'Hi, oh you're a nurse, what hospital do you work in?'

Make a list of the places where nurses work.

What skills do you think a nurse needs to do the job effectively, safely and compassionately?

How do you manage your time?

You may be given the outcome of your interview there and then. Some universities take longer to inform you of their decision; your offer will always be conditional on:

- an acceptable occupational health screen,
- a satisfactory criminal records check,
- suitable references.

Other conditions may apply; for example, you may have to achieve certain grades in specific subjects. You may be allowed to commence the programme on the understanding that you meet these conditions, and be asked to leave if you don't. It is your responsibility to meet the conditions.

SECTION SUMMARY

If you have not already applied to and been interviewed for a nursing programme you should go back over this section again and think about each subsection carefully, and how you will respond during the application process and when you attend for selection. Failure to adhere to the requirements or to meet the selection criteria will result in your application being rejected. You should always remember that the selection process is a two-way process and you are also assessing the university to determine whether it meets your needs.

Starting nurse education

Congratulations! You have been offered a place on your chosen programme in your chosen field. This is going to be the first day of the rest of your life.

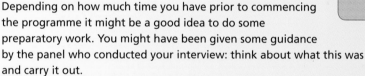

PEARLS OF WISDOM

Depending on how much time you have prior to commencing the programme it might be a good idea to do some preparatory work. You might have been given some guidance by the panel who conducted your interview: think about what this was and carry it out.

The programme you are about to embark on is going to be both intellectually and physically stimulating. If you do not do so already then start reading the broadsheet newspapers, particularly the health and social care sections. This will inform you about contemporary health and social care issues, and it can also improve your vocabulary.

If the opportunity arises and you are given the chance to work in a health or social care setting (paid or unpaid) then make the most of this: it will give you valuable work experience.

There are several weekly or fortnightly nursing journals available that you should read. This will offer an insight into some of the contemporary issues impacting on care delivery.

Meet other nursing, health and social care students.

ACTIVITY 1.2

Think of a nurse. What images came to mind?
- The sex object
- The buxom blonde
- The battleaxe
- An angel
- A gay man
- The murderer
- The professional
- The doctor's handmaiden

What do you think about this statement: 'No, I couldn't be a nurse, all that blood'.

Think about this statement: 'It doesn't matter if the nurse is male or female so long as they do their job well.' What are your comments?

Why are stereotypes damaging to the nursing profession?

How can negative stereotypes be changed?

Nursing is another branch of medicine: discuss.

How does the following statement make you feel? 'I am just a nurse.'

Do you want to fit the commonly held stereotype of a nurse or do you want to help change that stereotype?

I qualify at the end of this year. It's been hard work but worth it. I can't say I have enjoyed all of it but, I am really glad I did it. *Third year learning disabilities student*

You have come this far and now the next steps are ensuring that you get through the programme having developed the skills and qualities required to care for people safely, competently and compassionately.

Nursing provides a varied, challenging and rewarding career to those who would like to make a difference to the lives of people who live locally, nationally and internationally. Nurses are responsible for the care they provide and they have to answer for their own judgements, actions and omissions: this is called being accountable.

 ## Summary

To conclude this chapter the reader should look back to the quote at the beginning: nursing is the best job in the world. To undertake nursing education you really do have to want to do it: the work of the nurse is so varied and each day really is so different, but you only get out of it what you put into it. The roles and functions of the nurse have changed and will continue to change, and there are a number of career opportunities available to you in the UK and internationally once you have completed your programme and registered with the NMC.

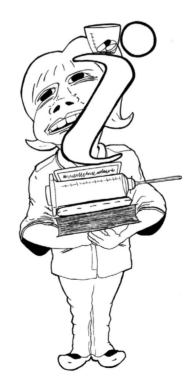

There are many really important things to consider prior to making your application for a place at a university. Think about the field of nursing you want to apply for, weigh up the pros and cons associated with the various universities and always remember that this is a two-way process: does that university offer you what you want? Becoming familiar with the entry criteria and the selection processes can help you progress onto a programme of study: aim to be selected, not rejected.

 # Resources

Bursary Administration Unit Northern Ireland
www.delni.gov.uk
Offers various types of funding support for the individual, employer or training organisations.

NHS Student Awards Wales
www.wales.nhs.uk/sitesplus/829/page/36092
The NHS Wales Student Award Unit implements the NHS Wales Bursary Schemes, which provides funding for healthcare students on NHS-funded courses in Wales.

NHS Student Grants Unit England
www.nhsbsa.nhs.uk/Students/3259.aspx
Provides all the information needed when applying for an NHS Bursary in England.

Students Awards Agency for Scotland
https://www.saas.gov.uk/student_support/special_circumstances/nursing_midwifery.htm
A Scottish Government agency, paying grants and bursaries to Scottish students in higher education.

UCAS (Universities and Colleges Admissions Service)
www.ucas.com/students/choosingcourses/specificsubjects/nursing
UCAS is the organisation responsible for managing applications to higher education courses in the UK.

CHAPTER 2

The Nursing and Midwifery Council and Other Regulatory Bodies

WHAT THIS CHAPTER CONTAINS

- Health profession regulation
- A discussion concerning the role and function of the Health and Care Professions Council (HCPC) and the General Medical Council (GMC)
- The role and function of the Nursing and Midwifery Council (NMC)
- The code of professional conduct
- The student's code

Health profession regulation

The provision of health and social care across the UK is regulated by a number of different organisations that work in a variety of different ways. There are some regulators, such as the Care Quality Commission in England or the Regulation and Quality Improvement Agency in Northern Ireland, that are responsible for checking the quality and safety of services. The Medicines and Healthcare Products Regulatory Agency, for example, works on the quality and safety of medicines and medical devices.

The Professional Standards Authority for Health and Social Care (PSA) aims to promote the health, safety and well-being of patients and other members of the public as well as independently promoting the voice for patients in the regulation of health professionals throughout the UK. Until December 2012 the PSA was known as the Council for Healthcare Regulatory Excellence (or CHRE).

The Student Nurse Toolkit: An Essential Guide for Surviving Your Course, First Edition. Ian Peate.
© 2013 John Wiley & Sons, Ltd. Published 2013 by John Wiley & Sons, Ltd.

ACTIVITY 2.1

If you were asked to put together a set of values and principles that would underpin an organisation that had the responsibility for regulating health and social care professionals, what would they be?

The values and principles of the PSA act as a framework for decision making.

The values of the PSA

- patient- and public-centred,
- independent,
- fair,
- transparent,
- proportionate,
- outcome-focused.

Its principles are:

- proportionality,
- accountability,
- consistency,
- targeting,
- transparency,
- agility.

Understanding the role and function of the various regulatory bodies can help you ensure that the care you provide to people is benchmarked against the standards that have been set. The PSA oversees the nine health professional regulators:

1 General Chiropractic Council (GCC),
2 General Dental Council (GDC),
3 General Medical Council (GMC),
4 General Optical Council (GOC),
5 General Osteopathic Council (GOsC),
6 General Pharmaceutical Council (GPC),
7 Health and Care Professions Council (HCPC),
8 Nursing and Midwifery Council (NMC),
9 Pharmaceutical Society of Northern Ireland (PSNI).

It oversees the activities of these professional regulators to ensure the promotion of the health, safety and well-being of patients and the public. It does this by:

- setting the standards of behaviour, competence and education that health professionals must meet,
- dealing with concerns from patients, the public and others about health professionals who are unfit to practise because of poor health, misconduct or poor performance,

- keeping registers of health professionals who are fit to practise in the UK,
- the regulators can remove professionals from their registers and prevent them from practising if they consider this to be in the best interests of the public.

The PSA has legal powers to:

- check how well the health professional regulators carry out their work,
- audit the initial handling of fitness-to-practise cases,
- refer cases to court where decisions are considered too lenient,
- give advice on policy.

It does this through:

- involving patients and the public in its work,
- promoting good practice,
- influencing national and international policy on health professional regulation,
- communicating with its stakeholders.

ACTIVITY 2.2

Go to the PSA website (www.professionalstandards.org.uk/home) and download its annual Performance Review Report. Here you will find a review undertaken by the PSA concerning key issues that affect health professional regulation which in turn can have the potential to impact on public protection. The performance review is the PSA's annual check on how effective the professional regulators have been in their role in protecting the public and promoting confidence in health professionals and themselves. The PSA is obliged to report its findings to Parliament and to the devolved administrations.

 ## The Health and Care Professions Council

The HCPC, like the NMC, is a regulatory body but whereas the NMC regulates two professions, nurses and midwives, the HCPC has responsibility for regulating 15 health professions (see Table 2.1). The General Social Care Council (GSCC) has been abolished. This provided the regulation of social workers in England and, from July 2012, has now become the responsibility of the renamed Health and Care Professions Council (HCPC).

The HCPC maintains a register of properly qualified health professionals for the public to check who meet HCPC standards for training, professional skills and good practice. Each of these professions has at least one professional title that is protected by law, including those shown in Table 2.1. This would mean, for example, that anyone using the titles 'physiotherapist' or 'dietitian' must be registered with the HCPC.

It is a criminal offence for anybody to say that they are registered with the HCPC when they are not.

Table 2.1 The professional bodies regulated by the HCPC

Profession	Role
Arts therapist	An art, music or drama therapist encourages people to express their feelings and emotions through art, such as painting and drawing, music or drama.
Biomedical scientists	Biomedical scientists analyse specimens from patients to provide data to help nurses, doctors and other healthcare professionals diagnose and treat disease.
Chiropodist/ podiatrist	A chiropodist/podiatrist diagnoses and treats disorders, diseases and deformities of the feet. They also work to promote good health and prevent disease.
Clinical scientist	A clinical scientist oversees specialist tests for diagnosing and managing disease. They offer advice to nurses, doctors and other healthcare professionals on using tests and interpreting data and they also carry out research to understand diseases and devise new therapies.
Dietitian	Dietitians use the science of nutrition to devise eating plans for patients to treat medical conditions. They also work to promote good health, helping to facilitate a positive change in food choices among individuals, groups and communities.
Hearing aid dispenser	Hearing aid dispensers work in private practice and assess, fit and provide aftercare in the dispensing of hearing aids. They also work to promote good health and prevent disease.
Occupational therapist	Occupational therapists use a number of activities to limit the effects of disability and promote independence in all aspects of daily living.
Operating department practitioner	Operating department practitioners participate in the assessment of the patient prior to surgery and provide individualised care in a number of settings.
Orthoptist	An orthoptist specialises in diagnosing and treating visual problems involving eye movement and alignment. They also work to promote good health and prevent eye disease.
Paramedic	Paramedics offer specialist care and treatment to people who are acutely ill or injured. They can administer a range of drugs and carry out certain surgical techniques.
Physiotherapist	Physiotherapists deal with human function and movement and help people to achieve their full physical potential. They use physical approaches to promote, maintain and restore well-being.
Practitioner psychologist	Psychologists work with people to attempt to understand the role of mental functions in individual and social behaviour.

Profession	Role
Prosthetist/othotist	Prosthetists and orthotists have responsibility for all aspects of supplying prostheses and orthoses for patients. A prosthesis is a device that replaces a body part that is missing. An orthosis is a device fitted to an existing body part with the intention of improving its function or to reduce pain.
Radiographer	Therapeutic radiographers plan and deliver treatment using radiation; for example, cancer treatments. Diagnostic radiographers produce and interpret high-quality images of the body with the intention of diagnosing injuries and diseases. For example, X-rays, ultrasound or CT scans carried out in hospital.
Speech and language therapist	Speech and language therapists assess, treat and help to prevent speech, language and swallowing difficulties.

ACTIVITY 2.3

You are caring for a child of 10 years old who has been diagnosed with paraganglioma (also called a glomus tumour) and has undergone surgical removal of this tumour. From the list in Table 2.1 what role would the healthcare professionals have in the care and treatment of this child? Would they all be involved in this person's care and treatment?

The duties of HCPC registrants are outlined in their code of conduct (Health Professions Council, 2004). Each registrant must confirm that they have read and agree to adhere to the standards described in the HCPC's *The Standards of Conduct, Performance and Ethics*.

Nurses work in teams and with a number of other health and social care workers and as such you need to know their various roles and functions. Understanding each other's role can help to enhance the patient experience and above all ensures that care delivery is safe and effective. Working as a team helps clinicians and patients put the pieces of the jigsaw together: making sense of the bigger picture can set the direction.

The General Medical Council

Another statutory body, the General Medical Council (GMC), an organisation independent of the NHS and of Government, has responsibility for maintaining the medical register for the UK. Just as the NMC has statutory powers, statutory powers under the UK Medical Act 1983 allow the GMC to take action where there are concerns about the fitness to practice of a registered medical practitioner (likewise, the General Dental Council regulates dentists and dental nurses).

If the GMC determines that a doctor is not fit to practise, it has powers to erase that doctor's name from the medical register (striking off), to suspend the doctor from the register or to place conditions on the doctor's practice. These actions are applicable to practice in any sector of employment in any part of the UK.

The GMC publishes the duties of a doctor registered with the GMC (General Medical Council, 2006). This guidance outlines the principles and values on which good practice is based, describing good medical professionalism in action.

The role and function of the Nursing and Midwifery Council

The Nursing and Midwifery Council (NMC) does not advocate for or represent nurses: this is undertaken by the unions. The NMC's role as regulator is to protect the public through the setting of standards and the regulation of those who are on the professional register. The titles nurse, midwife and health visitor are protected in law.

The NMC and its predecessor bodies have been in existence since 1919. The NMC is the regulator for the largest group of healthcare professionals, as there are 660 000 registered nurses and midwives. Like its predecessors the General Nursing Council (GNC) and the UK Council for Nursing, Midwifery and Health Visiting (UKCC), the NMC has a statutory duty to set standards and regulate the nursing, midwifery and health visiting professions. The NMC was established under the Nursing and Midwifery Order 2001 and came into being on 1 April 2002. It is accountable, through the Privy Council, to Parliament and members of the public.

The NMC's key purpose is to safeguard the health and well-being of the public and this is enshrined in law in the Nursing and Midwifery Order 2001. This aspect of law (and other associated elements of legislation) governs the work of the NMC. The NMC carries out a number of statutory obligations, which means that much of its work (its duties) has been set out in law.

The various pieces of legislation that direct and guide nurses and nursing can be confusing. Trying to make sense of them all can take some time.

The NMC:

- registers all nurses and midwives, ensuring that they are properly qualified and competent to work in the UK,
- sets the standards of education, training and conduct that nurses and midwives require in order to deliver high-quality healthcare consistently throughout their professional careers,
- ensures that all nurses and midwives keep their skills and knowledge up to date and uphold the standards of their professional code,

- ensures that midwives are safe to practise by setting rules for their practice and supervision,
- has fair processes in place to investigate allegations made against nurses and midwives who may not have followed the code.

The NMC regularly consults with nurses on issues that will have a direct or indirect impact on the profession, providing those nurses who wish to voice their opinions with the opportunity to do so. The NMC communicates with registrants and the public in a variety of ways. Its website contains much information that is easily accessible, aiming to ensure that everyone on the register is kept up to date about the new standards and guidance, information about current and upcoming consultations, details about new activities and initiatives and how they will affect nurses, as well as an assortment of other relevant information.

The NMC also communicates with registrants through its publication *NMC Review*, as well as communicating directly when necessary. For example, it contacted every nurse on the professional register to inform them of the various ways in which they could, if needed, raise and escalate concerns regarding care (whistleblowing).

SECTION SUMMARY

Ensuring the safety of the public is a common theme associated with all bodies that regulate health and social care professionals. Most professional regulators produce codes of professional conduct (standards) as well as maintaining a professional register. Provision is in place to address issues associated with allegations of professional misconduct.

 Education and conduct

Standards for education and conduct are also set by the NMC with the aim of ensuring that nurses have the appropriate skills and qualities when they commence work. The previous sentence mentions two important things: skills and qualities. The skills you require as a nurse to carry out your job effectively are multifaceted, encompassing interpersonal skills and technical skills. Both are required to ensure safe, effective care: they are called psychomotor skills.

 I was learning how to draw up an injection, it looked so easy on television, on *Casualty*. I didn't just need an extra pair of hands to draw up the fluid, get the dose right, be sure it was the right drug, maintain sterility, make sure I was safe and didn't stab anyone – I needed to be an octopus, this was such a difficult procedure.
First year adult student nurse

The technical skills that are required to draw up an injection are essential, so too are the interpersonal skills. The nurse needs to communicate effectively to ensure that the patient is safe and understands the reason for the injection and the potential side effects, and to give consent.

Performing effectively means that the nurse has to perform to the standards set by the NMC and the NMC makes known these standards through the *Code* (Nursing and Midwifery Council, 2008; more about this in the next section).

 Managing concerns and allegations

Another important function of the NMC is the management of concerns or allegations that may have been made about a nurse, midwife or health visitor. If an allegation has been made about a nurse whereby it is felt that the NMC's standards for skills, education and behaviour have not been met, or that there is a problem with the nurse's work, the NMC has to carry out an investigation. If needed, it will act by removing the nurse from the register, either permanently or for a specific period of time.

PEARLS OF WISDOM

Think always of the person you are caring for first and foremost. With this at the front of your mind you are well on the way to ensuring that your practice is patient-centred. Using the evidence to guide your thoughts and deeds provides the person with safe and effective care.

Never, ever, be afraid to say 'I don't know'. Acknowledging your limitations is not a sign of weakness or deficiency; it is your way of saying, I am here to protect the people I care for and I do not wish to do them any harm intentionally or unintentionally.

If you are unsure then ask; nobody will mind you asking questions. In fact, it is expected that you ask questions, seek clarification and do the right thing. There are many people who you can turn to for help and advice while on placement (wherever that may be) or in the university.

 The *Code*

The Code: Standards of Conduct, Performance and Ethics for Nurses and Midwives (shortened to the *Code*; Nursing and Midwifery Council, 2008) is a key tool in safeguarding the health and well-being of the public. It is the foundation on which good nursing practice is based and applies to all registered nurses and midwives. The opening lines of the *Code* states that:

> The people you care for must be able to trust you with their health and well-being.

The *Code* was first published in 2008 and is subject to change and reform as time passes. The *Code* should not be seen as a stick with which to beat registrants (those nurses on the professional register). It should be used as a tool for nurses to enhance and promote safe and effective nursing care. The *Code* is written with input from nurses in the four countries of the UK, along with other stakeholders including service users.

SECTION SUMMARY

The NMC's code of professional conduct provides registrants and the public with an outline of the standards expected of those whose name appears on the professional register. Failure by the nurse to adhere to the tenets enshrined within the *Code* can lead to an investigation of any shortfalls.

 ## Professional conduct: student nurses

Often members of the public cannot distinguish students from qualified nursing staff. It is essential that students uphold the reputation of the profession: while studying as well as in their personal lives. The NMC has produced guidance on professional conduct for nursing students (Nursing and Midwifery Council, 2010) based on the strict standards laid out in the *Code* (Nursing and Midwifery Council, 2008). The aim of this guidance is to help students act with integrity and to work or emulate working in a professional manner as they prepare to enter the profession that brings with it great privileges and responsibilities. It helps student nurses demonstrate fitness to practise. The guidance provides information to students concerning:

- the role of the NMC,
- good health and good character,
- behaviour and conduct,
- the code of professional conduct,
- asking for help.

As well as the guidance produced by the NMC your own university will also provide you with advice about the standards expected of you during the 3 years of your course. Most universities also provide an overview of your privileges as a student with the intention of helping you succeed in your studies.

This is often produced in the form of a students' charter and is usually adapted specifically for students who are studying health and social care-related programmes due to the unique relationship such students have with the people in their care.

ACTIVITY 2.4

Search for the students' charter of your own university and think about its contents. You may see information concerning;
- attendance,
- what to do when off sick (in placement or when at university),
- the provision of support,
- issues concerning equal opportunities,
- respect for each other,
- harassment and bullying,
- making appeals,
- conduct and behaviour.

Then compare this with the NMC's guidance on professional conduct for nursing students. There will be many similarities and a number of health and social care-specific issues, such as health and safety, and personal safety while on placement.

Nursing students are not the only students who have a student code. Go to the General Pharmaceutical Council website (www. pharmacyregulation.org/sites/default/files/Code%20of%20conduct%20 for%20phamacy%20students%20s.pdf). Here you will find the *Code of Conduct for Pharmacy Students*; again, compare and contrast this with the NMCs guidance.

> I was a first year student working in a hospital in Staffordshire. The standard of care was so bad I agonised for days – should I say something or not? Eventually I did. I spoke to the link teacher; he was great made me feel safe and I thought if I feel safe so too should the patients. I was petrified, but it was absolutely the right thing to do. *Belinda, third year adult student*

Being aware of the various codes of conduct, the many regulatory bodies and the requirements demanded by your university can help ensure that you are starting your nursing career with the intention of becoming a professional and a highly skilled practitioner. The codes of conduct provide you with guidance and describe the standards required.

Good health, good character and fitness to practise

The Nursing and Midwifery Council (2010) provides guidance on good health, good character and fitness to practise (Chapter 1 of this book also addresses these issues). To practise as a nurse effectively, safely and without supervision you must have good health. A number of people with a disability and long-term health conditions are practising, some of whom need reasonable adjustment and some of whom do not; therefore, good health is more than the absence of any disability or health condition.

Just as important is good character; the public must be assured that nurses are honest and trustworthy. Good character incorporates issues such as a person's behaviour and their attitude. The NMC also take into account and consider any convictions or cautions that are not deemed compatible with your role as a registered nurse or that may bring the profession into disrepute. Character must be considered sufficiently good for the nurse to be capable of providing safe and effective care without supervision.

Having the appropriate skills knowledge, good health and good character to offer safe and effective care is associated with fitness to practise. Throughout your nursing education you will be assessed continually in association with your fitness to practise. Any concerns arising about this will be investigated and addressed by the university.

Each university implements its own processes associated with good health, good character and fitness to practise. Some universities do this annually.

 ## Summary

The public deserve to be cared for by nurses who have demonstrated that they are safe and effective. This is also true of other health and social care professionals; for example, social workers, paramedics, pharmacists and doctors.

The activities of regulatory bodies such as the NMC, HCPC and GMC are overseen by the PSA, which has a number of powers enabling it to ensure that the health and social care regulators are doing their job effectively.

A student's code of conduct in the form of guidance has been produced by the NMC and addresses important issues such as good health, good character and fitness to practise.

 ## References

General Medical Council (2006) *The Duties of a Doctor Registered with the GMC*. General Medical Council, London

Health Professions Council (2004) *The Standards of Conduct, Performance and Ethics*. Health Professions Council, London

Nursing and Midwifery Council (2008) *The Code: Standards of Conduct, Performance and Ethics for Nurses and Midwives*. Nursing and Midwifery Council, London

Nursing and Midwifery Council (2010) *Guidance on Professional Conduct for Nursing and Midwifery Students*, 2nd edn. Nursing and Midwifery Council, London

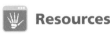

Resources

Professional Standards Authority for Health and Social Care

www.professionalstandards.org.uk/home

The PSA oversees nine health professional regulators, promoting the health, safety and well-being of patients and the public. They have number of powers allowing them to check how well the regulatory bodies carry out their work

General Medical Council

www.gmc-uk.org/

Registers doctors to practise medicine in the UK. Protecting, promoting and maintaining the health and safety of the public by ensuring proper standards in the practice of medicine.

Health and Care Professions Council

www.hpc-uk.org/

A professional regulator set up to protect the public. The HCPC keeps a register of health professionals who meet its standards for training, professional skills, behaviour and health.

National Union of Students

www.nus.org.uk/

The NUS is a voluntary membership organisation. It is a confederation of 600 students' unions, amounting to more than 95% of all higher and further education unions in the UK. It represents the interests of more than 7 million students.

Nursing and Midwifery Council

www.nmc-uk.org/

The nursing and midwifery regulator for England, Wales, Scotland, Northern Ireland and the Islands. It exists to safeguard the health and well-being of the public and set standards of education, training, conduct and performance. The NMC ensures that nurses and midwives keep their skills and knowledge up to date and uphold professional standards.

Royal College of Nursing

www.rcn.org.uk/

The RCN represents nurses and nursing, promotes excellence in practice and shapes health policies; it is the biggest professional union for nurses in the UK. The RCN support students throughout their studies, providing representation associated with your rights, and offering advice and other services. RCN students are actively encouraged to voice their opinions and they can do this through the RCN Student Discussion Zone.

UNISON

www.unison.org.uk/

UNISON is the UK's largest public service union, representing more than 1.3 million people providing vital services to the public. UNISON has more than 25000 student nurse members, dedicated to campaigning for a better deal for nursing and midwifery students, running several campaigns around areas such as the bursary and accommodation.

CHAPTER 3

Nursing Education: the Standards for Pre-registration Nurse Education

WHAT THIS CHAPTER CONTAINS

- A brief history of nurse education
- An overview of the standards for pre-registration nurse education

The quality of nursing in the UK is an issue of great public focus and concern. What nurses do and how they have been educated and prepared to carry out their role raises much interest from many parties. Nurses and nursing have been and will continue to be under constant examination by the public and the media.

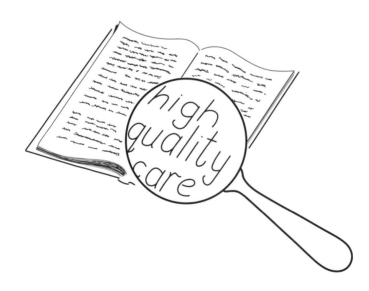

The Student Nurse Toolkit: An Essential Guide for Surviving Your Course, First Edition. Ian Peate.
© 2013 John Wiley & Sons, Ltd. Published 2013 by John Wiley & Sons, Ltd.

Nursing is dynamic, and the Royal College of Nursing (2003) define it as:

> the use of clinical judgement in the provision of care to enable people to improve, maintain or recover health, to cope with health problems, and to achieve the best possible quality of life, whatever their disease or disability until death.

Nurses practice nursing in a range of settings from acute hospital trusts to people's homes, schools and other places. It has been well recognised for some time that nurses are and always will be the pivot on which the NHS turns. Nurses should never be seen as doctors' handmaidens. The contribution nurses make to the health and well-being of people is phenomenal; nurses possess their own unique knowledge base and their own individual skills that go towards ensuring that their work and the work of the multidisciplinary team is effective, with the patient at the heart of all they do.

ACTIVITY 3.1

Before you read any further in this chapter, devise a job description for a newly qualified staff nurse. Choose any area of care (e.g. community or hospital) and field of nursing. You might want to consider the Royal College of Nursing's definition of nursing to help you. Keep this until you get to the end of this chapter and then revisit the job description and see if there are any changes you would like to make to it in light of having read about nursing curricula, the new Nursing and Midwifery Council standards and public interest.

The term pre-registration nursing education refers to the programme that a nursing student in the UK commences with the requirement of acquiring the competencies necessary to meet the criteria for registration with the NMC.

 At that time I was a first year, first-warder and I was on a male orthopaedic ward and was petrified when I walked on the ward for the first time. I couldn't even spell the word orthopaedic, the nurses all seemed to know what they were doing and I was sure I was in the way. After a few weeks I really settled in and at the time decided I wanted to work in orthopaedics, the job just seemed to be so varied. I am being interviewed for a staff nurse's job on an orthopaedic ward next week: fingers crossed.
Chris, third year adult student (now a staff nurse)

A brief history of nurse education

In 1858 state registration had begun for the medical profession. Support for the regulation of nursing became more common after organised nurse training was established in 1860. This was the year that Florence Nightingale opened the Nightingale Training School for Nurses at St Thomas' Hospital, London. The intention was to train nurses to a qualified and specialised level, with the key aim of learning to develop observation skills and sensitivity to the needs of patients. After this the trainee nurses were allowed to work in hospitals across the UK and abroad. This first school allowed the training of nurses to flourish and now nursing is taught at a number of British and other universities.

Nightingale was not a supporter of any form of regulation for nursing; it was her belief that the important qualities of the nurse could not be taught, examined or regulated. Ethel Bedford Fenwick, one-time Matron of St Bartholomew's Hospital, London, was keen to unite all British nurses in membership of a recognised profession, as evidence of their having received systematic training.

In 1902 the Midwives Registration Act established the state regulation of midwives. It was the First World War that provided the final incentive to the establishment of nursing regulation. A Private Member's Bill was introduced to establish a regulatory system and was eventually passed in December 1919, and separate Nurses Registration Acts were passed for England and Wales, Scotland and Ireland (which at that time was still a single country). The General Nursing Council for England and Wales and the other bodies were established by this Act until changes in the law occurred in 1979 and the UK Central Council for Nursing Midwifery and Health Visiting (UKCC) and the national boards were created.

The Briggs Committee was set up in 1970 to consider issues concerning the quality and nature of nurse training as well as the place of nursing within the NHS, and in 1972 chair Asa Briggs released the Briggs Report. The committee made a number of recommendations associated with changes to professional education. In 1979, after 6 years of debate and delay, the Nurses, Midwives and Health Visitors Act 1979 was passed and a number of changes were made to regulatory structures, including the establishment of a unified central council and separate boards in each of the four countries with particular responsibility for education.

The influential Briggs Report and the Nurses, Midwives and Health Visitors Act 1979 paved the way for Project 2000. This was implemented in 1989, and under it new students commenced their nurse education programme together, by undertaking a common 18-month foundation programme, and then branched into the branches of child, mental health, adult or learning disabilities (this was later changed to a 1-year common foundation programme and a 2-year branch). This marked a decisive break with the familiar apprenticeship style of nursing training (Bradshaw, 2001). Schools of Nursing moved from their sites in NHS hospitals to the higher education setting, but the programmes remained 50% theory and 50% practice. The new learner was to be seen as a knowledgeable doer who would be research-aware and research-capable.

The UKCC was set up in 1983 and its core functions were to maintain a register of UK nurses, midwives and health visitors, offer guidance to registrants and manage professional misconduct complaints. At the same time, national boards were created for each of the UK countries. Their key activity was to monitor the quality of nursing and midwifery education courses, and to maintain the training records of students on these courses.

The UKCC ceased to exist in April 2002 and its functions were taken over by the current Nursing and Midwifery Council (NMC). The activity undertaken by the four national boards were also brought to an end and quality assurance functions associated with education were adopted by the NMC (Ousey, 2011).

In 2009 the NMC announced that by 2013 the minimum academic award for all pre-registration nursing programmes would be at degree level (Nursing and Midwifery Council, 2009). The introduction of new standards for pre-registration nursing education (Nursing and Midwifery Council, 2010a) has been the biggest shake-up for nurse education in decades.

SECTION SUMMARY

Nurse education, over the centuries, has changed constantly; originally religious orders took on responsibility for helping to train novices to tend to the sick and dying. Nightingale was responsible for the more formal type of training with similarities seen around the world even today. In the UK, with formalised training came regulation. The apprentice type of education used in the UK for many years has now been replaced by degree-level study.

 ## Standards for pre-registration nurse education

The NMC describes a standard as something that will be fully met only when all the requirements have been demonstrated. Normally this occurs during the validation process as well as during the NMC's annual review of programmes of study, but the NMC monitor and will seek reassurance with regards to quality as and when they see fit. Guidance issued by the NMC, on the other hand, is something that they view as good practice and which should be followed. There is some flexibility in how guidance is applied to education programmes. If there is evidence that it is not followed precisely, the programme provider (your university) will have to account for this, explaining how an alternative approach will produce a similar outcome.

ACTIVITY 3.2

Rank the following publications by the NMC as guidance or standards.

	Tick: guidance or standard?	
	Guidance	Standard
The *Code*		
Medicines management		
Record keeping		
Midwives rules		
Supervised practice of midwives		
Care of older people		
Raising and escalating concerns		
Proficiency for specialist community public health nurses		

A review and consultation were undertaken by the NMC during 2007 and 2008 in relation to the principles for pre-registration nurse education. The review had two phases, examining what future nurse education would need to look like to enable nurses to meet the needs of patients safely and efficiently. The first phase reviewed the principles of a future framework and the next phase developed the standards that would support the framework. Over 5000 individuals and organisations contributed to the review.

PEARLS OF WISDOM

Take time to understand the NMC standards as well as the nursing curriculum that your university is working with. This is important as it will allow you to understand why you are doing what you are doing; it will also enable you to take more responsibility for your learning. Understanding the content of the curriculum can help you make decisions about your education in a more effective manner. Even better, get involved in curriculum-development activities at your university; this allows you to put your point across as well as the views of fellow students. You can add to your CV that you were part of the curriculum-development team ensuring that standards for education and practice were fit for purpose and of a high quality.

Eight confirmed principles were agreed to support a new framework for pre-registration nursing education (Nursing and Midwifery Council, 2009).

Principle 1: academic level

(i)   The minimum award for pre-registration nursing programmes in the UK is nursing registration with a degree; meeting the programme hours is European Directive 2005/36/EC.
(ii) There are no opportunities to register as a nurse if a degree cannot be achieved.

Principle 2: professional recognition

(i)   Registration on the nursing part of the register with a mark denoting one field of practice, in: adult, children's, mental health or learning disability nursing.
(ii) Modernised pathways leading to registration as a nurse in each of these four fields of practice.

Principle 3: nature of programme

(i)   Preparation is characterised by a blend of generic (see note) and field-specific learning, extending throughout the programme with the field-specific component growing over time (*note*: generic refers to a whole class or group, as opposed to specific individuals or subgroups, i.e. for the whole of nursing rather than a nursing field).
(ii) Flexible boundaries between the generic and field-specific components with extensive opportunities for shared learning.
(iii) Specified NMC competencies for (a) generic and field-specific practice, (b) community and public health practice and (c) European Union requirements for general care (adult field).
(iv) NMC outcome measures linked to progression points.

Principle 4: length of programme

(i)   Minimum of 3 years, or 4600 hours, full-time or part-time equivalent (to be completed in 5 years full time, or 7 years part time).
(ii) Fifty per cent theory to practice ratio.
(iii) Combination of both community and other practice learning sufficient to achieve required outcomes.

Principle 5: integrated care pathways and themes

(i)   The ways in which care pathways and themes used to organise healthcare in respective countries are incorporated into the curriculum is for local determination.

Principle 6: stepping on

(i) Maximum of 50% accreditation of prior (experiential) learning (AP(E)L) linked to progression points subject to requirements of European Directive 2005/36/EC.

Principle 7: recognition when stepping off a programme early

(i) Transcript to quantify theory and practice achievement.

Principle 8: period after registration

(i) Mandatory preceptorship to follow initial registration.

See Table 3.1 for the four fields of nursing.

Table 3.1 The fields of nursing

Field	Activity
Adult	The focus of care is generally on the provision of care for people aged over 18 years who are ill, recovering from an accident or illness or learning to live with a disability.
Mental health	Mental health nursing offers care to people of all ages; this includes children who may be experiencing or who may be at risk of developing mental health problems. Care provision can focus on supporting people's physical, psychological, social, mental and spiritual health and recovery needs.
Learning disability	Care is provided to people of all ages and includes those children who have learning disability; the aim is to maximise the person's health and independence. Nurses work closely with families and careers offering care and advice with regards to meeting challenging and complex needs.
Children	Children's nurses provide care to children and young people from birth to mid to late teens in a number of community and hospital care settings. Partnership working is a key feature of children's nursing working with children, young people and their families.

Source: adapted from Nursing and Midwifery Council (2010a, 2010b).

The need for new standards for pre-registration nursing education

Healthcare is changing and in response to this new standards for pre-registration nursing education have been introduced. Care provision will increasingly be provided in the community or closer to home rather than in hospitals; life expectancy has risen and continues to increase and health needs are becoming frequently more complex (see Chapter 4 in this book). The role of the nurse has been extended and nurses have increasingly specialist roles and the authority to prescribe medicines, and they use the latest practices and techniques to meet complex clinical needs. Changes to the way pre-registration education progammes have been delivered will enable future nurses to meet these increasing demands.

ACTIVITY 3.3

It has been said that an increase in life expectancy is a factor that was considered when the new standards were developed. Can you think of other factors that would have been taken into consideration to ensure that nursing curricula are fit for purpose?

 ## The new standards and service provision

The introduction of the standards and service provision has provided employers (service providers) with an opportunity to review their future nursing workforce and ensure that newly qualified nurses are fit for purpose and able to provide care that will be rated by service users as excellent.

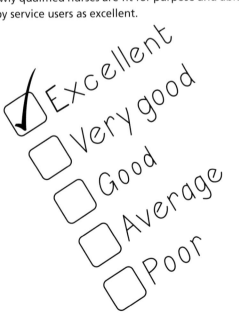

The move to degree-level education as the foundation for professional nursing will continue to prepare the next and future generations of nurses to be able to care for people safely and effectively. Employers have been involved in evaluating the current overarching programme (most universities will have two programmes running simultaneously: those using the old standards (proficiencies) and those using the new standards (competencies)). This has allowed successful aspects of previous approaches to be carried over and areas for improvement to be identified while developing new curricula. There is much emphasis in the new standards on partnership working between employers and education providers: curricula have been jointly developed. The aim was to ensure that programmes met the requirements for the student to gain NMC registration but also educated graduates to become fit for employment. Strong partnership working will result in practice learning opportunities that reflect the content of the curriculum and thus the student experience is maximised.

During the development process opportunities for practice learning outside of traditional settings were provided, making sure that the learning needs of the programme and the preparation of students for delivering healthcare in a different way were offered. More and more healthcare is being delivered in a wider range of settings, caring for and treating people with complex health issues where people will have a greater say and choice over their own healthcare.

To be sure that the newly registered nurse is fit for purpose and has the ability to practice in any environment where care is provided, now and in the future, students need to be exposed to more non-traditional learning opportunities (Chapter 8 discusses practice learning opportunities in more detail): these opportunities should be of high quality and innovative.

The NMC (Nursing and Midwifery Council, 2010b) suggests that those nurses who are educated to degree level will be able to offer better care, they will be able to:

- practise independently, making autonomous decisions,
- think analytically, using higher levels of professional judgement and decision making in complex care settings,
- plan, deliver and evaluate effective, evidence-based care safely and with confidence,
- offer complex care using state-of-the-art technology,
- drive up standards and quality,
- manage resources, work across service boundaries,
- lead, delegate, supervise and challenge other nurses and healthcare professionals,
- lead and participate in multidisciplinary teams,
- provide leadership in promoting and sustaining change and innovation.

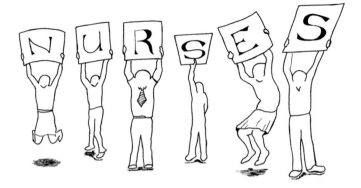

66 I am just about finishing my programme, I will graduate with
a diploma not a degree but, I will be working with the same
university to top up to a degree over the next year or so. *Churchill,
third year student* 99

SECTION SUMMARY

The new standards for nurse education were developed
by a wide range of stakeholders and this included NHS,
independent and third-sector representation. It was essential
that the stakeholders engaged with the development of the standards
to ensure they were fit for purpose and practice. There has been a move
from traditional practice placements to more innovative placements for
students, providing the staff nurse of tomorrow with insight into and
hands-on experience of the many locations where health and social care
is delivered.

The standards for education

The standards for education provide the mandatory requirements in which you
must be deemed competent before you will be admitted to the professional
register: the point of registration. The new requirements have come from a variety of sources including previous rules, standards and guidance, and key policies
from the four UK Government health departments, as well as conforming to the
relevant European Union directives and guidelines. The new standards will eventually replace the 2004 standards (Nursing and Midwifery Council, 2004).

The standards exist to ensure that you will be able to function safely and effectively in the future, responding to the needs of growing and complex health and
social care systems, so that you can care for people in a variety of venues, working

flexibly as a member of the multidisciplinary team. Those who are able to demonstrate that they have met the mandatory standards and have the appropriate knowledge, skills and behaviours will be equipped to improve health and wellbeing, and undertake a variety of roles, including:

- ๐ practitioner,
- ๐ educator,
- ๐ manager,
- ๐ leader,
- ๐ researcher.

The standards contain the requirements and guidance that all universities or other approved education institutions (AEIs) and their partners (for example, those in the NHS) within the UK must adhere to in the development and delivery of education programmes.

As the role of the nurse continues to develop and become more and more diverse, programmes of study that prepare nurses to gain entry to the professional register must also be dynamic and flexible enough to ensure that student nurses are fit for purpose and can start lifelong careers once their educations conclude.

The pre-registration programme of study that prepares nurses for registration with the NMC has also developed over the years; most recently this has been with regards to the introduction of new standards.

Standards for competence

The competency framework provides the standards for competence and the related competencies that all nursing students must acquire prior to applying to be registered at first level on the nurses' part of the professional register.

The programme of study must take no less than 4600 hours over a minimum of 3 years and you must complete it within 5 years or, if the programme is offered part time, 7 years. There is a requirement that 50% of the programme is practice-based for you to gain the required practical knowledge, skills and behaviours in a number of care environments working with a variety of people and their families with various levels of dependency. The remaining half of the programme is spent in the educational establishment (the university) and you are expected to acquire the theory needed to support your practice enabling the competencies to be achieved.

Each university is given autonomy to design its own nursing curriculum; the NMC does not have a national curriculum. Any curriculum that seeks to prepare nurses to have their name entered on to the professional register must be able to demonstrate that the nurses they are preparing will be able to deliver care with competence and confidence wherever they practise, to a range of people with various needs. All curricula undergo an NMC validation event, which assesses and assures quality.

NMC quality assurance

ACTIVITY 3.4

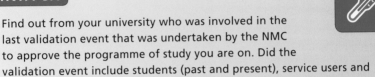

Find out from your university who was involved in the last validation event that was undertaken by the NMC to approve the programme of study you are on. Did the validation event include students (past and present), service users and qualified nurses?

The term competence used by the NMC is derived from the Queensland Nursing Council (Queensland Health, 2009) and is defined as a holistic concept that requires the learner to combine and demonstrate their knowledge base, their skill acquisition, values, beliefs, attitudes and technical ability when delivering care in a safe and effective manner.

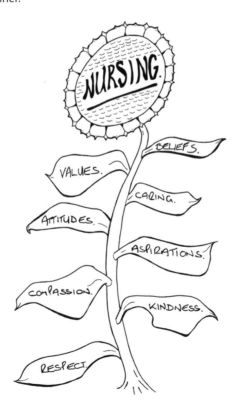

The competencies are set out under four domains:

1 professional values,
2 communication and interpersonal skills,
3 nursing practice and decision making,
4 leadership, management and team working.

Each domain is generic in nature as well as having a field-specific attribute. Table 3.2 provides an example of the domain of professional values with an example of the generic and four field-specific attributes.

You may have noticed in this standard that much of it is derived from the NMC code of conduct (Nursing and Midwifery Council, 2008a). It is essential therefore that you fully understand what the *Code* contains and how it will guide and influence the way you progress on your programme of study.

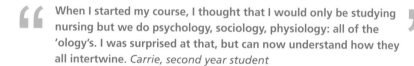

When I started my course, I thought that I would only be studying nursing but we do psychology, sociology, physiology: all of the 'ology's. I was surprised at that, but can now understand how they all intertwine. *Carrie, second year student*

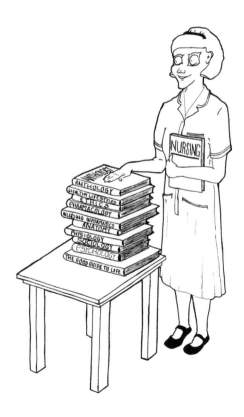

Table 3.2 The professional values domain describing the generic and field- specific standards

Generic standard for competence: professional values
All nurses must act first and foremost to care for and safeguard the public. They must practise autonomously and be responsible and accountable for safe, compassionate, person-centred, evidence-based nursing that respects and maintains dignity and human rights. They must show professionalism and integrity and work within recognised professional, ethical and legal frameworks. They must work in partnership with other health and social care professionals and agencies, service users, their carers and families in all settings, including the community, ensuring that decisions about care are shared.

Field-specific standard for competence: professional values

Adult	Children's	Learning disabilities	Mental health
Adult nurses must also be able at all times to promote the rights, choices and wishes of all adults and, where appropriate, children and young people, paying particular attention to equality, diversity and the needs of an ageing population. They must be able to work in partnership to address people's needs in all healthcare settings.	Children's nurses must understand their role as an advocate for children, young people and their families, and work in partnership with them. They must deliver child and family-centred care; empower children and young people to express their views and preferences; and maintain and recognise their rights and best interests.	Learning disabilities nurses must promote the individuality, independence, rights, choice and social inclusion of people with learning disabilities and highlight their strengths and abilities at all times while encouraging others to do the same. They must facilitate the active participation of families and carers.	Mental health nurses must work with people of all ages using value-based mental health frameworks. They must use different methods of engaging people, and work in a way that promotes positive relationships focused on social inclusion, human rights and recovery; that is, a person's ability to live a self-directed life, with or without symptoms, that they believe is meaningful and satisfying.

Source: Nursing and Midwifery Council (2010a).

 ## Standards for education

There are 10 standards for education and these standards must be met for pro-gramme approval and ongoing delivery. They form a framework within which your programme is delivered, they also specify the requirements that all programmes

must meet, including those that relate to the teaching, learning and assessment of nursing students, conforming with the NMC's standards to support learning and assessment in practice (Nursing and Midwifery Council, 2008b). Box 3.1 lists the 10 standards for education.

Box 3.1 The 10 education standards

1. Safeguarding the public
2. Equality and diversity
3. Selection, admission, progression and completion
4. Support of students and educators
5. Structure, design and delivery of programmes
6. Practice learning opportunities
7. Outcomes
8. Assessment
9. Resources
10. Quality assurance

Source: Nursing and Midwifery Council (2010a).

If you look closely at your own programme structure you should be able to pick out the 10 standards for education.

 ## Summary

Nurse education, like the provision of health and social care, is not static and has not been so since Nightingale opened her first school of nursing in 1860. The preparation of healthcare professionals, including nurses, must continue to evolve to keep pace with the many rapidly changing biological, sociological and technological changes in health and social care.

You need to understand how the programme you are on was devised, the drivers that have impacted on how it was eventually structured and how you are being assessed and why. This chapter has provided you with some insight into the NMC's standards for registration nursing education. You are encouraged to delve deeper and to become involved in curriculum design and development.

 ## References

Bradshaw, A. (2001) *The Project 2000 Nurse*. Whurr, London

Nursing and Midwifery Council (2004) *Standards of Proficiency for Pre-registration Nursing Education*. Nursing and Midwifery Council, London

Nursing and Midwifery Council (2008a) *The Code: Standards of Conduct, Performance and Ethics for Nurses and Midwives*. Nursing and Midwifery Council, London

Nursing and Midwifery Council (2008b) *Standards to Support Learning and Assessment in Practice*. Nursing and Midwifery Council, London

Nursing and Midwifery Council (2009) *Confirmed Principles to Support a New Framework for Pre-registration Nursing Education.* www.nmc-uk.org/Get-involved/Consultations/Past-consultations/By-year/Pre-registration-nursing-education-Phase-1-/Confirmed-principles-to-support-a-new-framework-for-pre-registration-nursing-education/

Nursing and Midwifery Council (2010a) *Standards for Pre registration Nursing Education.* http://standards.nmc-uk.org/PublishedDocuments/Standards%20for%20pre-registration%20nursing%20education%2016082010.pdf

Nursing and Midwifery Council (2010b) *Pre Registration Nursing Education in the UK.* http://standards.nmc-uk.org/Documents/Pre-registration%20nursing%20education%20in%20UK%20FINAL%2006092010.pdf

Ousey, K. (2011) The changing face of student nurse education and training programmes. *Wounds UK* 7(1), 70–6

Queensland Health (2009) *Community Health Nursing, Competency and Skills.* Queensland Health, Townsville Health Services District, Queensland

Royal College of Nursing (2003) *Defining Nursing.* Royal College of Nursing, London

 ## Resources

NHS Employers

www.nhsemployers.org/PlanningYourWorkforce/Nursing/nursingeducationandtraining/PreRegistration/Pages/Implementingthepre-registrationstandards-gettingstarted.aspx

NHS Employers exists to help employers make sense of current and emerging healthcare issues, collecting and analysing the views of employers and using contacts and opportunities to ensure that the voice of employers is heard in the fast-moving health-reform agenda. This website specifically addresses issues and concerns associated with implementation of the NMC's standards for pre-registration nursing.

Nursing and Midwifery Council

www.nmc-uk.org/

See Resources section in Chapter 2

Royal College of Nursing

www.rcn.org.uk/

See Resources section in Chapter 2

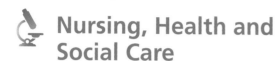

CHAPTER 4

Nursing, Health and Social Care

WHAT THIS CHAPTER CONTAINS

- ☙ A discussion on care delivery and key drivers
- ☙ Health and social care
- ☙ Issues related to the vulnerable patient
- ☙ How to raise and make known your concerns

Chapter 3 describes some of the ways in which nursing education across the UK has had to transform and respond to changing needs, developments, priorities and expectations in health and healthcare. This chapter builds upon the previous chapters and discusses healthcare delivery systems and the way they work and will have to work to meet present and future challenges, improve health and well-being and to drive up standards and quality.

ACTIVITY 4.1

Have look at the short video clip, *Smile*, a commercial from an NHS nursing recruitment campaign. The commercial is the NHS's most successful direct response campaign and recorded over 90 000 replies in 6 weeks. See it at www.youtube.com/watch?v=lryyTgNlR1w.

The video clip demonstrates the range of services the public can expect to receive from the NHS. The NHS was set up in 1948 to offer care free at the point of use, a comprehensive and universally national system, and it has become the world's largest publically funded health service. The provision of health

---

The Student Nurse Toolkit: An Essential Guide for Surviving Your Course, First Edition. Ian Peate.
© 2013 John Wiley & Sons, Ltd. Published 2013 by John Wiley & Sons, Ltd.

and social care is expensive, contrary to the belief that healthcare is free in the UK. The provision of health and social care takes up a large proportion of the taxpayer's money and also attracts much media attention. Spending on health and social care accounts for £1 in every £10 of the UK's gross domestic product (GDP), more than £150 billion a year. The NHS employs more than 1.7 million people across the UK (Naylor and Appleby, 2012). Despite these large sums of money being spent on health and social care financial problems and inequalities in funding still exist.

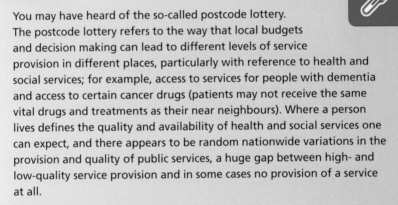

ACTIVITY 4.2

You may have heard of the so-called postcode lottery. The postcode lottery refers to the way that local budgets and decision making can lead to different levels of service provision in different places, particularly with reference to health and social services; for example, access to services for people with dementia and access to certain cancer drugs (patients may not receive the same vital drugs and treatments as their near neighbours). Where a person lives defines the quality and availability of health and social services one can expect, and there appears to be random nationwide variations in the provision and quality of public services, a huge gap between high- and low-quality service provision and in some cases no provision of a service at all.

Think of the following:

access to services for people with dementia,
access to treatments and drugs for some forms of cancer.

How might service provision differ across the four countries of the UK and also within the four countries?

What impact might this have on those people and their families needing those services?

Activity 4.2 points out that the gap between the values associated with a comprehensive and universal 'national' health service and reality is being increasingly stretched. Ways in which health and social care are provided require reform. This variation between healthcare provision (including the quality of care), infection rates, referrals, treatment options and waiting times, for example, exacerbates inequalities and social exclusion.

SECTION SUMMARY

Millions of people come into contact with health and social care systems and often it is the nurse who is at the centre of all of this and who is seen as the coordinator of care. Billions of pounds are spent each year on providing people with care and health services and, as ever, health and social care systems are changing and will continue to change with the intention of providing safe and cost effective care. There are a number of inequalities in health and social care provision and the changes ahead will go some way to ensuring that the inequalities in provision of services are a thing of the past.

 # Healthcare

It is the state, to a large extent, that accepts much responsibility for the health of its populace; there are usually three key ways in which healthcare is funded:

- tax-based funding,
- state insurance,
- private insurance.

The tax-based model is the one that is generally used in the UK, with an increase in the engagement of the non-statutory (voluntary) and private (independent) sectors offering more provision related to health and social care services (see Chapter 2 for a discussion on regulation).

Health is a concept that is often difficult to define, as each person may have their own definition of what health means depending on their own unique and individual circumstances. The World Health Organization (1948) provided a definition of health:

A state of complete physical, mental and social well-being and not merely the absence of disease.

This definition offers a positive approach to health, focusing on biological, psychological social aspects of the being. However, it must be remembered it may not fit with everybody's own personal definition of health.

Healthcare provision can be divided into three (see Table 4.1). The differences between primary, secondary and tertiary care are blurring with an increased emphasis on care being provided close to the person's home, in the community (Department of Health, 2006). Service provision has traditionally been defined by the professions, which have shaped services to reflect their own speciality, areas of expertise and interests. This is changing. More emphasis is now being placed on what the patients say they want and what their preferences are; the concept of the 'expert patient' has been gaining momentum. The patient often knows more about their condition than the healthcare provider as they learn to cope with their often long-term condition.

Table 4.1 Healthcare provision: primary, secondary and tertiary

	Primary	Secondary	Tertiary
	Care provided by practice nurses, GPs and other professionals in practices, clinics and community settings, such as the person's home	Care provided in an acute care setting such as: acute trusts, ambulance trusts, mental health trusts or care trusts	Specialised centres offering care associated with very complex conditions
Services	Preventative services such as immunisations and the offer of screening programmes (cervical screening) Care provision, for example changing dressings, minor surgery, providing treatment such as prescriptions and drug administration	The provision of elective or emergency care. In elective care, care is planned and requires specialist services or surgical intervention. Often admission to secondary care occurs following referral from a primary or community health professional such as a practice nurse or GP. Care can be offered on an outpatient basis.	Patients are usually inpatients requiring specialist care and may be referred by a primary or secondary health professional, to a service that has staff and facilities for advanced medical investigation and treatment. Tertiary care services include cancer management, neurosurgery, cardiac surgery, plastic surgery, treatment for severe burns, advanced neonatology and palliative care.

ACTIVITY 4.3

How are long-term conditions defined?

Make a list of all the long-term conditions you can think of. Now marry that list (if you can) with voluntary or charitable organisations that exist to help those people and their families manage that condition. Some examples are given on the table to start you off.

Long-term condition	Voluntary (charitable) organisation
Asthma	Asthma UK
Sickle cell disease	Sickle Cell Society

The patient is now becoming increasingly seen as a partner in their care; indeed, the principle of 'no decisions about me without me' was central to recent UK Government health and social care reforms (Department of Health, 2010a). The principle describes a vision of health and social care where the patient is listened to, and is an equal partner as well as an active participant in treatment decisions (Department of Health, 2010b).

It is estimated that there are over 7 million carers in Britain (Baggot, 2012). People are increasing their use of self-help and self-medication (for example, seeking over-the-counter medications) and those with long-term chronic conditions are self-managing their health and their illness. These countervailing forces are challenging the status quo and traditional approaches to healthcare provision and the management of healthcare.

Social care

Social care is an essential human need and is something many of us will need at some point in our lives, possibly for ourselves or those who are close to us. How well we look after each other says a great deal about the strength and character of our society (Department of Health, 2010a).

Social care has its origins in nineteenth-century philanthropy (Glasby, 2012). The provision of social care in the UK has changed many times over the years with a number of key drivers forcing these changes. The Beveridge Report published in 1942 (Beveridge, 1942) makes reference to the five giant evils facing society at that time; Lord Beveridge's report formed the basis for much of today's social legislation (see Table 4.2).

It is essential, according to Glasby (2012), to make the distinction between several key terms; often these terms are used interchangeably. 'Social care', he suggests, is an overall description for a range of services and workers who support both adults and children who face challenges in their lives; the services are provided by

Table 4.2 A comparison between Beveridge and contemporary welfare services

The five giant evils	Current comparison
Want	Social security
Disease	NHS
Ignorance	Education/lifelong learning
Squalor	Housing/regeneration
Idleness	Employment/leisure

Source: adapted Glasby (2012).

a number of providers. This broad description has had a focus on providing practical support for a number of specific service user groups, and these include children at risk of abuse, older people who are at risk, those people with mental health problems, people with learning difficulties and people who are disabled.

It has been estimated that there are over 1.6 million people using social care services and 1.4 million people working in the social care workforce: this is more than the entire NHS workforce. Social care staff are employed by 30 000 public, private and voluntary organizations and the services spend in the region of around £16 billion per year. It must be noted here that there are many people using social care services who are funding their own care.

A social worker is a degree-trained professional registered with a formal council (the Health and Care Professions Council, HCPC) who like nurses are governed by a code of professional conduct. They typically care and work with people who have been socially excluded or who are experiencing crisis across the public, private and voluntary sectors. A key role is the provision of support to enable service users to help themselves; while maintaining professional relationships with service users social workers act as guides, advocates or critical friends.

Social workers work in a number of settings within a framework of relevant legislation and procedures, supporting individuals, families and groups within the community; these may include the service user's home, schools, hospitals or the premises of other public sector and voluntary organisations. Registered social work professionals are often supported by social work assistants, working closely with other health and social care staff.

> At our university we have social work students who are working towards their degree and we have to shadow one of them for a week. It was so good to be able to see how other professionals work and what their work entails. The social work course is a tough course. *Jasmina, second year learning disabilities student*

Social work and social workers are central to the Government's vision for a modern system of social care. The Department of Health (2010a) suggests that the vision is to be built on seven principles, as follows.

1 Prevention: empowered people and strong communities will work together to maintain independence. Where the state is needed, it supports communities and helps people to retain and regain independence.
2 Personalisation: individuals, not institutions, take control of their care. Personal budgets, preferably as direct payments, are provided to all eligible people. Information about care and support is available for all local people, regardless of whether or not they fund their own care.
3 Partnership: care and support delivered in a partnership between individuals, communities, the voluntary and private sectors, the NHS and councils, including wider support services, such as housing.
4 Plurality: the variety of people's needs is matched by diverse service provision, with a broad market of high-quality service providers.
5 Protection: there are sensible safeguards against the risk of abuse or neglect. Risk is no longer an excuse to limit people's freedom.
6 Productivity: greater local accountability will drive improvements and innovation to deliver higher productivity and high-quality care and support services. A focus on publishing information about agreed quality outcomes will support transparency and accountability.
7 People: we can draw on a workforce who can provide care and support with skill, compassion and imagination, and who are given the freedom and support to do so. We need the whole workforce, including care workers, nurses, occupational therapists, physiotherapists and social workers, alongside carers and the people who use services, to lead the changes set out here.

This new vision, the new model, stresses greater choice and control, enhanced partnership working and more emphasis on citizenship and social inclusion. There is a pressing need to refocus service provision to adopt a preventative approach with more interagency working, with the service user at the centre.

> I was asked if I wanted to sit in on a case meeting (a kind of conference) concerning a lady with a profound mental health condition; the idea was to discuss her care plan. The lady was present with her friend and a number of other healthcare professionals. I was so anxious but the way all of the people there worked together with this woman really brought home the importance of working together with the best interests of patients as central. *Jerry, first year, first ward mental health student*

Just as the health services face challenges in the twenty-first century so too do the social services: there is an ageing population, medical and technological advances, and changes in family availability to offer support. All of this is associated with a range of social, economic and demographic changes. To cope and manage with these profound changes there is a need for closer partnership working.

Partnership working

The provision of effective health and social care systems depends on a number of other services, such as social care, transport, and housing. The close working relationship with these other services has not always been as effective as it could have been in the past (of course, there are some exceptions), and in particular those who provide social care services. There are a number of reasons why these services have not worked as well as they could; for example, organizational and cultural differences associated with NHS and local government.

There have been a number of laudable efforts to address these problems, including joint planning and the setting up of joint financial arrangements, the introduction of 'pooled budgets' between local authorities and the NHS, and a closer alignment of local authority boundaries with Primary Care Trusts. However, there is still a need to make more effort in joining up and providing the service user with a seamless service; the NHS and local authorities have to work more closely.

☀ Health and social care reform

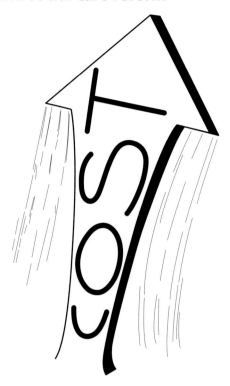

The NHS (particularly in England, but not exclusively) is undergoing much reform, and all of this is taking place against a background of global economic austerity (HM Government, 2010). Changes and reorganisation are made in an attempt to promote and provide a more consistent service. There will be more emphasis on improving cost-effectiveness; interventions must be able to demonstrate efficacy and quality-enhancing technologies will be introduced (this will also include improved information technology systems).

Major reforms to the NHS in England have been proposed by the Government. The White Paper *Equity and Excellence: Liberating the NHS*, published in July 2010 (Department of Health, 2010a), set out plans to give more power to patients and health professionals. Following royal assent the Health and Social Care Bill became the Health and Social Act 2012. It is difficult to predict what impact the new Act will have on patients, service users and carers (including nurses).

Key issues will focus upon the integration of health and social care services with the intention of:

- ☍ strengthening patient and public involvement in health,
- ☍ increasing accountability,

☵ enabling good monitoring and scrutiny,

☵ providing patients and the public real influence on commissioning decisions.

In April 2013 the commissioning of services underwent radical change and Primary Care Trusts and Strategic Health Authorities were abolished as part of a radical structural reorganisation, with new Health and Wellbeing Boards established to improve integration between the NHS and local authority services. Around 2000 clinical commissioning groups now have the responsibility for commissioning and will work with the new NHS Commissioning Board. It is anticipated that these groups will take control of 60% of the NHS budget and enable general practitioners, with the support of other clinicians and managers, to decide how best to meet the needs of the local populations they serve.

There is a new regulator called Monitor and its role will be to regulate providers of NHS services in the interests of patients and help ensure that anticompetitive behaviour is prevented. Monitor will license providers of care and identify at an early stage whether a provider is at risk; for example, because of financial difficulties. All NHS providers will become Foundation Trusts by 2014 and it will become easier for private and third-sector organisations to enter the market. It is thought the plurality of healthcare provision will encourage innovation and creativity, by encouraging competition between the NHS, the private sector and the voluntary sector.

The voice of patients has been strengthened through the setting up of a new national body, Healthwatch, along with local Healthwatch organisations. Healthwatch will play a significant role at both the national and local levels, ensuring that the views of the public and those who use the services are taken into account.

Public health has also undergone significant changes. Nationally, Public Health England has been established to work across government on health improvement, and local authorities have taken charge of public health responsibilities at a local level. Funding for public health has been transferred from the NHS to local authorities in line with these changes, with the expectation that local authorities will work closely with NHS organisations in discharging their new duties.

As time passes it is important to remember that often a gap exists between policy intent and what actually happens in practice. With regards to health and social reforms experience has demonstrated that there are many challenges associated with the conversion of bold aspirations into action and it may take many years to see those aspirations come to fruition.

PEARLS OF WISDOM

It is essential that you work with other healthcare providers to ensure that you respect the impact that their contribution has made on the overall care experience. There is no place in contemporary health and social for provision rivalry: the focus of care should centre on the patient and not on the various healthcare professionals.

SECTION SUMMARY

It was the aim of the Health and Social Care Act 2012 to enable nurses and doctors to tailor services for patients, to offer more choice to patients over how they are treated and to reduce bureaucracy in the NHS. The Act has:

- devolved power to front-line nurses and doctors: health professionals are free to design and tailor local health services for their patients;
- driven up quality: patients will benefit from a renewed focus on improving quality and outcomes;
- ensured a focus on the integration of services: there will be strong pressure on the health service to promote integration of services;
- strengthened public health: giving responsibility for local public health services to local authorities will ensure that they are able to pull together the work done by the NHS, social care, housing, environmental health, leisure and transport services;
- given patients more information and choice: patients now have greater information concerning how the NHS is performing and the range of providers they can choose for their healthcare; they have a stronger voice through Healthwatch England and local Healthwatch;
- strengthened local democratic involvement: power has moved from central government to town halls and there will be at least one locally elected councillor and a representative of Healthwatch on every Health and Wellbeing Board, with the intention of influencing and challenging commissioning decisions and to promote integrated health and care;
- reduced bureaucracy: two layers of management – Primary Care Trusts and Strategic Health Authorities – have been removed through the Act, resulting in a saving of £4.5 billion.

The implementation of the Act has enabled patients, clinical leaders (nurses and doctors), patients' representatives and local government to take new and leading roles in shaping more effective services.

The vulnerable person

Amidst all of the changes and the various attempts to integrate service provision is the patient, the person services are provided for. There are times when people, for a number of reasons, become vulnerable. A vulnerable adult is defined as:

> A person over 18 years of age who may be in need of community care services by reason of mental or other disability, age or illness; and who is or may be unable to protect him or herself against significant harm or exploitation (Department of Health, 2000).

There are six principles associated with safeguarding adults (Department of Health, 2011), as listed below.

Principle 1. Empowerment: presumption of person led decisions and consent

Principle 2. Protection: support and representation for those in greatest need

Principle 3. Prevention: prevention of harm and abuse is a primary objective

Principle 4. Proportionality: proportionality and least intrusive response appropriate to the risk presented

Principle 5. Partnerships: local solutions through services working with communities

Principle 6. Accountability: accountability and transparency in delivering safeguarding

All those who provide health services have a duty to safeguard all patients as well as providing further measures for those patients who are less able to protect themselves from harm or abuse. Each individual has a right to live a life that is free from harm and abuse; this is an absolute fundamental human right and is an essential requirement for health and well-being. Nurses often work with patients who for a number of reasons may be less able to protect themselves from neglect, harm or abuse.

The concept of 'safeguarding' adults addresses a wide spectrum of activity from prevention through to multiagency responses where harm and abuse have occurred. A multiagency approach and procedures must apply where there is concern of neglect, harm or abuse to a patient defined as vulnerable.

There are some concerns that may appear minor in nature but which provide an opportunity for early intervention, such as advice to prevent a problem escalating. Other safeguarding concerns can be more serious and may require a response through multiagency procedures and possible statutory intervention through health and social care regulators, the criminal justice system or civil courts.

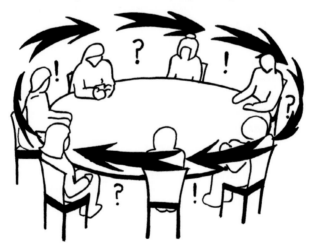

Harm and abuse can be physical, sexual, psychological, discriminatory, financial or neglectful in nature. It may involve a one-off incident or can be extensive across a service.

Harm or abuse can occur in a variety of settings, such as within regulated services and in people's own homes. Likewise, the cause of harm and abuse may also be wide-ranging; for example, harm caused unintentionally by an unsupported carer, neglect caused by staff or a service or abuse that is caused through thoughtlessness or is intentional.

The Nursing and Midwifery Council (2009) provides some examples of abuse, including:

- physical: hitting, slapping, pushing or restraining,
- psychological: shouting, swearing, ignoring, blaming or humiliating,
- sexual: forcing a person to take part in any sexual activity without their consent,
- financial and material: illegal or unauthorised use of someone's property, money or valuables, theft, fraud,
- neglect: depriving a person of food, clothing, heat, comfort, stimulation or essential care,
- acts of omission: failing to provide medication or treatment, or omitting essential aspects of care.

If you have any immediate concerns regarding abuse these must be dealt with under local safeguarding policies and procedures in the first instance. The National Patient Safety Authority (2009) has provided information that may help you if you have concerns or worries about patient safety incidents.

Speaking out

Safeguarding adults is a key element of patient care and the duties required to safeguard patients are laid down by professional regulators and service regulators, and are supported in law. You must make known your concerns in an appropriate manner; this includes using local policies, clinical governance and risk-management processes. Report your concerns to the appropriate person or authority immediately if you suspect or see potential risk to the safety of those you care for, if there is immediate risk or harm, then report these concerns at once.

Sometimes it is not always so easy to speak out; for example, you may not know how to go about doing this, you might be scared of reprisals and you could even feel that you are being disloyal. This can be exacerbated further if you are working alone or if you work in remote, small communities. At all times you must remember that the person you are caring for is your first concern: you must never forget this. If you raise an issue early then this can prevent them from becoming more serious, causing more harm to the person or people being cared for.

It is acknowledged that it can be uncomfortable for you if you are feeling intimidated or isolated but there is help at hand that you can use for guidance and support if you are ever feeling unsure. For example:

- your tutor,
- your mentor/facilitator,
- your trade union (for example, UNISON),

⚕ your professional body (for example, the Royal College of Nursing),

⚕ the charity Public Concern at Work (an independent whistleblowing charity).

All of the above can raise issues formally and may be able to act for you on your behalf; they can also provide you with personal support.

As an advocate one part of your work is to speak up for the people you care for: it is unacceptable to do nothing. When you raise concerns and speak up this shows that you are dedicated to the people for whom you care. Figure 4.1 outlines the stages for raising concerns.

PEARLS OF WISDOM

Silence is not golden.

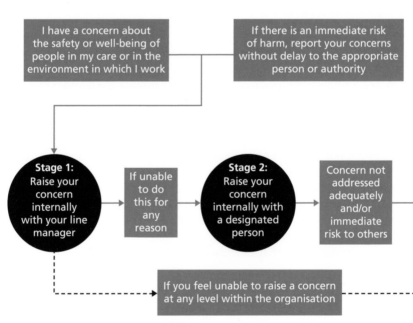

Figure 4.1 Stages for raising and escalating concerns. *Independent, confidential advice is available from your professional body, trade union or Public Concern at Work (see Resources). Students can also speak to their university tutor, lecturer or mentor.
Source: Nursing and Midwifery Council (2010).

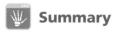 **Summary**

Care-delivery systems have changed, are changing and will continue to change and there are a number of key drivers associated with these changes. Hospitals and health and social care sectors will be challenged by several major trends in the future. Some examples are listed here.

- The ageing population will increase the level of care required by patients, having an impact on hospitals, nursing homes and the provision of care in the person's home.
- Lifestyle diseases are global problems and as the rate of critical and chronic lifestyle diseases increases the hospital and healthcare sectors will be challenged, having to care for increasing numbers of patients.
- As global economies fluctuate spending reforms are in force, with the possibility of compromising further investment in health and social care.
- The worldwide obesity phenomenon, a result of changing lifestyles, is placing a further burden on overstretched hospital and healthcare sectors.

Health and social care reforms aim to put in place systems and processes that will allow the health and social care sectors to manage the changes ahead with the patient at the centre of all that is done. The changes ahead present both a challenge and an opportunity to all healthcare professionals and providers.

Society has a duty to protect the vulnerable and in terms of health and social care this means that people must be protected from harm. Vulnerability can occur at any time and all nurses must be alert to the signs that abuse has happened or is going to happen. Early intervention can prevent harm occurring. Knowing how to escalate concerns is an important aspect of the role and function of the nurse.

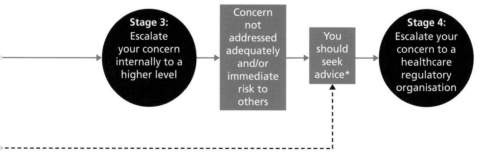

References

Baggot, R. (2012) Health care. In Alcock, P., May, M. and Wright, S. (eds), *The Student's Companion to Social Policy*. Wiley, Oxford, pp. 331–7

Beveridge, W. (1942) *Report of the Inter-Departmental Committee on Social Insurance and Allied Services*. HMSO, London

Department of Health (2000) *No Secrets; Guidance on Development and Implementing Multi-Agency Policies and Procedures to Protect Vulnerable Adults form Abuse*. Department of Health, London

Department of Health (2006) *Our Health, Our Care, Our Say: A New Direction for Community Services*. Department of Health, London

Department of Health (2010a) *Equity and Excellence: Liberating the NHS*. Department of Health, London

Department of Health (2010b) *A Vision for Adult Social Care: Capable Communities and Active Citizens*. Department of Health, London

Department of Health (2011) *Safeguarding Adults: The Role of Health Service Practitioners*. Department of Health, London

Glasby, J. (2012) Social care. In Alcock, P., May, M. and Wright, S. (eds), *The Student's Companion to Social Policy*. Wiley, Oxford, pp. 359–65

HM Government (2010) *Spending Review 2010*. The Stationery Office, London

Naylor, C. and Appleby, J. (2012) *Sustainable Health and Social Care. Connecting Environmental and Financial Performance*. Kings Fund, London

National Patient Safety Authority (2009) *Being Open: Communicating Patient Safety Incidents with Patients, Their Families and Carers*. www.nrls.npsa.nhs.uk/resources/?entryid45=65077

Nursing and Midwifery Council (2009) *Guidance for the Care of Older People*. Nursing and Midwifery Council, London

Nursing and Midwifery Council (2010) *Raising and Escalating Concerns. Guidance for Nurses and Midwives*. Nursing and Midwifery Council, London

World Health Organization (1948) *Preamble to the Constitution of the World Health Organization as Adopted by the International Health Conference*. New York, 19–22 June 1946, entered into force on 7 April 1948

 Resources

Carers Trust

www.carers.org/

The Carers Trust is a UK-wide trust that works to improve support, services and recognition for anyone living with the challenges of caring, unpaid, for a family member or friend who is ill, frail, disabled or has mental health or addiction problems. The trust's Network Partners aim to ensure that information, advice and practical support are available to all carers across the UK.

Carers UK

www.carersuk.org/

A charity set up to help the millions of people who care for family or friends. Carers UK provides information and advice about caring alongside practical and emotional support for carers. It also campaigns to make life better for carers and influence policy makers, employers and service providers, to help them improve the lives if carers.

Public Concern at Work

www.pcaw.org.uk/

Public Concern at Work is a whistleblowing charity. They offer free, confidential advice to people concerned about crime, danger or wrongdoing at work, help organisations to deliver and demonstrate good governance, inform public policy and promote individual responsibility, and organisational accountability in the public interest.

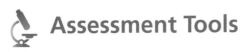
Assessment Tools

WHAT THIS CHAPTER CONTAINS

- ☼ An overview of the nursing process
- ☼ Waterlow pressure ulcer assessment tool
- ☼ Malnutrition Universal Screening Tool
- ☼ Modified Early Warning Score
- ☼ Glasgow Coma Scale

To care for people effectively you have to be able to apply a systematic approach to the care you deliver; otherwise it becomes ad hoc, disorganised and, in some cases, may be dangerous. The nursing process employs a systematic approach to care that helps you work through ways, using a cyclical method, in which to identify issues needing intervention. It is important to note that the process is cyclical as opposed to linear in nature.

The nursing process is used as a problem-solving framework when nurses plan and deliver care to patients (Burke *et al.*, 2011), and it can also help you prioritise patient care. If used appropriately the nursing process can be purposeful, with each of the steps designed in such a way as to achieve a specific purpose. The steps guide you to think systemically and in an organised manner, helping to prevent any omissions. The nursing process can have four to six phases associated with it (see Table 5.1). Regardless of the number of phases that are used this is a systematic, cyclical approach to care, as outlined in Figure 5.1.

As you become more skilled in using this tool your confidence and competence will grow and you will begin to develop new and innovative ways of helping people to resolve their problems and respond effectively to their needs. The nursing process can help you begin to think like a nurse, and it is the first tool that you will use to do this.

The Student Nurse Toolkit: An Essential Guide for Surviving Your Course, First Edition. Ian Peate.
© 2013 John Wiley & Sons, Ltd. Published 2013 by John Wiley & Sons, Ltd.

Table 5.1 The phases of the nursing process

Approach 1	Approach 2	Approach 3
1. Assessment	1. Assesssment	1. Assessment
2. Planning	2. Nursing diagnosis	2. Nursing diagnosis
3. Implementation	3. Planning	3. Outcome identification
4. Evaluation	4. Implementation	4. Planning
	5. Evaluation	5. Implementation
		6. Evaluation

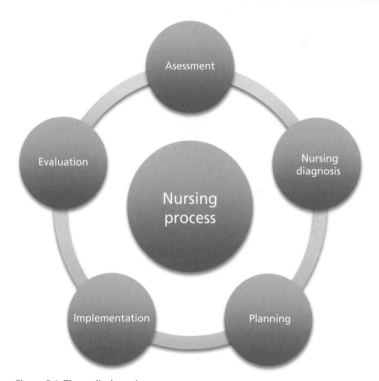

Figure 5.1 The cyclical nursing process.

 When I was a first year student and they spoke about this thing called the nursing process in class, its sounded so mysterious, the teacher said that we use processes every day in our lives and the nursing process is a process applied to nursing, and this really was the case. He was so right, the mystery was easier to deal with when explained in this way, now in my final year I am much more confident with it – not perfect, but getting there. *Femi, third year student*

ACTIVITY 5.1

Think purposely about a systemic approach to everyday life. Think about getting dinner ready for some friends. You need to apply the process.

Assess: how many people are you cooking for, what are their likes, dislikes, what budget do you have, what food do you already have in the house?

Diagnosis: this would be the type of food (the selection) you will serve to the people who are coming to dinner.

Planning: in this stage you have to plan the actual meal, work through a recipe maybe, so that it all comes together.

Implementation: the doing part of the meal, the cooking, getting the table ready and serving the meal, safely and effectively.

Evaluation: how did your guests find it; receiving their feedback. Did they enjoy it? Would you do anything different next time?

Think of some other activities, for example applying a systemic process to planning a holiday or travelling from point A to point B.

The nursing process underpins almost all nursing models used by nurses and also provides a tool for critical thinking and decision making.

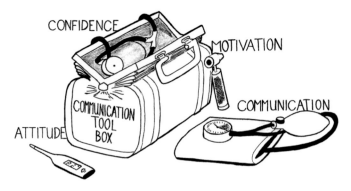

ACTIVITY 5.2

Who are the authors of the following models of nursing care?

Model	Author
Self Care Theory	
Activities of Living	
Adaptation Model	
Theory of Interpersonal Relations	

 The phases of the nursing process

Table 5.1 demonstrates that there can be anything from four to six stages or steps associated with the nursing process. A common approach is to use the five integrated steps approach. Table 5.2 provides a brief description of each step of the nursing process.

Table 5.2 A brief description of five steps associated with the nursing process

Step or phase	Brief description
Assessment	Collecting data about the health status of the patient; the data help to monitor for any evidence of health problems and potential risks to health. This stage allows you to begin to predict or detect.
Diagnosis	The analysis of the data collected enables you to draw conclusions and determine inferences. The diagnosis of patient problems are only possible once the nurse has gained sufficient experience and expertise; making a diagnosis independent of experience can be wrong and therefore potentially dangerous.
Planning	During this stage you now plan the care required to address the issues noted during assessment and the making of a diagnosis. You determine outcomes at this stage and identify appropriate interventions to achieve the outcomes. You set priorities that help detect further problems, and prevent and manage health problems and risk factors.
Implementation	Here you carry out what you planned in the previous stage: the plan of care is put into action, and you observe the response the patient is making to the care interventions.
Evaluation	Here you to undertake a comprehensive assessment of the patient to determine whether your actions have led to the expected outcomes, or whether new problems have emerged. The outcome of your comprehensive assessment may require you to modify or terminate the plan.

Each stage or phase of the nursing process is dynamic, fluid and often over-laps (see Figure 5.2). An accurate diagnosis will depend on an accurate assessment and accurate planning demands an accurate diagnosis. The planning stage guides interventions and is performed during the implementation stage. Evaluation is an important part of the implementation stage: as the nurse provides the care, the response that the patient is making to the interventions is being monitored, so that changes can be made as early as possible if necessary.

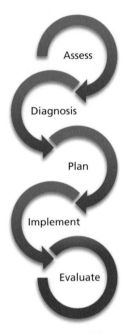

Figure 5.2 The integrated and overlapping phases of the nursing process.

SECTION SUMMARY

The nursing process (developed by Yara and Walsh, 1967) should be seen as a problem-solving approach whereby the nurse and the patient work together to assess needs, make a diagnosis, plan care, implement that plan of care and evaluate its effectiveness. The nursing process is a continuous, systematic and cyclical approach to the provision of care. Models of nursing are an essential element of the nursing process, helping guide the nurse to manage care.

Assessment tools

Assessment tools are designed to encapsulate a systematic approach to assessment but at the same time they recognise and embrace the nurse's professional decision making that occurs in the relationship between a nurse and another person. The nurse's professional judgement must always be used in determining the risk status of the patient; no risk-assessment tool can ever replace this.

Risk-assessment tools, for example those used to help nurses predict a patient's risk of falls, malnutrition and pressure ulcers, have been used extensively by nurses in a number of care areas. The tools have many uses, but they are only tools and should only be used to help make decisions and predict risk.

 ## The Waterlow pressure ulcer assessment tool

The Waterlow pressure ulcer assessment tool (see Figure 5.3) takes the assessment through stages, moving from a general 'narrative-based' assessment of 'domains' of care need to a more focused assessment of specific aspects of risk and complexity.

WATERLOW PRESSURE ULCER PREVENTION/TREATMENT POLICY
RING SCORES IN TABLE, ADD TOTAL. MORE THAN 1 SCORE/CATEGORY CAN BE USED

BUILD/WEIGHT FOR HEIGHT		SKIN TYPE VISUAL RISK AREAS		SEX AGE		MALNUTRITION SCREENING TOOL (MST) (Nutrition Vol.15, No.6 1999 - Australia			
AVERAGE BMI = 20-24.9	0	HEALTHY	0	MALE	1	A - HAS PATIENT LOST		B - WEIGHT LOSS SCORE	
ABOVE AVERAGE BMI = 25-29.9	1	TISSUE PAPER	1	FEMALE	2	WEIGHT RECENTLY		0.5 - 5Kg = 1	
		DRY	1	14 - 49	1	YES - GO TO B		5 - 10Kg = 2	
OBESE BMI > 30	2	OEDEMATOUS	1	50 - 64	2	NO - GO TO C		10 - 15 Kg = 3	
		CLAMMY, PYREXIA	1	65 - 74	3	UNSURE - GO TO C		> 15Kg = 4	
BELOW AVERAGE BMI < 20	3	DISCOLOURED GRADE 1	2	75 - 80	4	AND		unsure = 2	
BMI = Wt (Kg)/Ht (m)2		BROKEN/SPOTS GRADE 2-4	3	81 +	5	SCORE 2			
						C - PATIENT EATING POORLY OR LACK OF APPETITE 'NO' - 0, 'YES' SCORE - 1		NUTRITION SCORE If > 2 refer for nutrition assessment/intervention	

CONTINENCE		MOBILITY		SPECIAL RISKS					
COMPLETE/ CATHETERISED	0	FULLY	0	TISSUE MALNUTRITION		NEUROLOGICAL DEFICIT			
		RESTLESS/FIDGETY	1						
URINE INCONT,	1	APATHETIC	2	TERMINAL CACHEXIA	8	DIABETES, MS, CVA		4-6	
FAECAL INCONT,	2	RESTRICTED	3	MULTIPLE ORGAN FAILURE	8	MOTOR/SENSORY		4-6	
URINARY + FAECAL INCONTINENCE	3	BEDBOUND e.g. TRACTION	4	SINGLE ORGAN FAILURE (RESP, RENAL, CARDIAC,)	5	PARAPLEGIA (MAX OF 6)		4-6	
		CHAIRBOUND e.g. WHEELCHAIR	5	PERIPHERAL VASCULAR DISEASE	5	MAJOR SURGERY or TRAUMA			
SCORE				ANAEMIA (Hb < 8)	2	ORTHOPAEDIC/SPINAL		5	
10+ AT RISK				SMOKING	1	ON TABLE > 2 HR#		5	
15+ HIGH RISK						ON TABLE > 6 HR#		8	
20+ VERY HIGH RISK				MEDICATION - CYTOTOXICS LONG TERM/HIGH DOSE STEROIDS, ANTI-INFLAMMATORY MAX OF 4					

Scores can be discounted after 48 hours provided patient is recovering normally

© J Waterlow 1985 Revised 2005*
Obtainable from the Nook, Stoke Road, Henlade TAUNTON TA3 5LX
* The 2005 revision incorporates the research undertaken by Queensland Health.

Figure 5.3 The Waterlow pressure ulcer assessment tool. © Judy Waterlow, with kind permission. www.judy-waterlow.co.uk/.

The Waterlow score is one of a number of tools available to nurses that uses a numerical system to assess pressure ulcer risk. The various tools can help nurses identify patient needs and then act as a signpost to further needs. However, all risk-assessment tools have limitations (Griffiths, 2009), and this should always be borne in mind when using them.

ACTIVITY 5.3

This activity is designed to help you understand how to use a tool such as Waterlow (see Figure 5.3) and then assign an at-risk score to a patient, such as the one described below.

- Mrs Manpreet Saini is 67-year-old woman admitted to the nursing home where you work.
- Manpreet has type 2 diabetes.
- She has become unstable on her feet and is now finding it more difficult to get around without any help; her mobility has become restricted.
- Recently she has lost weight (12 kg), saying she has no appetite.
- On a number of occasions Mrs Saini has been incontinent of urine.
- Blood tests reveal she has an iron-deficiency anaemia.
- She has been prescribed a course of steroids.

Mrs Saini is now more dependent on others for her care needs. With this short patient history in mind calculate Mrs Saini's at-risk score using the Waterlow tool.

Once a nurse has conducted a full assessment of a patient using the Waterlow tool and applied clinical judgement, the next stage is to provide a plan of care and then implement it. This is to reduce the risks arising or to prevent deterioration of the current condition. For example, provision will need to be made to provide the patient with special pressure-relieving aids as well as to implement nursing-oriented activities such as frequent turning. The tool should be used on an ongoing basis so that care activities can be continually evaluated and new actions implemented should they be needed.

Malnutrition Universal Screening Tool

The Malnutrition Universal Screening Tool (MUST) is a nutritional risk-assessment tool using five stages to identify adults who are malnourished or at risk of malnutrition, including undernutrition and obesity. The British Association for Parenteral and Enteral Nutrition (BAPEN) has produced a MUST explanatory booklet (British Association for Parenteral and Enteral Nutrition, 2011) to help nurses use the tool to assess the patient, then plan and implement the appropriate care. The booklet has been formulated for use in hospitals, community and other care settings and has the advantage that it can be used by all care workers. The booklet explains the need for nutritional screening and how this can be undertaken using the MUST.

The five MUST steps (British Association for Parenteral and Enteral Nutrition, 2011) are as follows.

Step 1: gather nutritional measurements. Measure height and weight to obtain a body mass index (BMI) score (see below). If unable to obtain height and weight, then the nurse should use other alternative procedures.

Step 2: note the percentage of unplanned weight loss and score using tables that are provided in the tool kit.

Step 3: establish acute disease effect and calculate the score.

Step 4: add scores from steps 1, 2 and 3 together to obtain an overall risk of malnutrition.

Step 5: use management guidelines and/or local policy to develop a care plan.

The following formula is used to calculate a person's BMI manually:

$$BMI = \frac{\text{Weight in kilograms}}{\text{Height in metres, squared}}$$

There are three steps associated with this calculation.

1 Obtain height in metres and multiply the figure by itself.
2 Measure weight in kilograms.
3 Divide the weight by the height squared (this is the answer to the calculation in the first step).

For example, a patient might be 1.6 m tall and weigh 65 kg. The calculation would then be:

$$BMI = 65/(1.6 \times 1.6) = 65/2.56 = 25.39 \text{ kg/m}^2$$

A BMI calculator such as that shown in Figure 5.4 can also be used. The figure also shows the categories of body size. When the final score is obtained you can decide whether person falls into the underweight, normal, overweight or obese category.

ACTIVITY 5.4

Calculate the BMI for the patients in the table below and determine their nutritional health status, i.e. underweight, normal, overweight or obese.

Weight (kg)	Height (cm)	Nutritional status
80	163	
62	155	
49	170	
60	170	

Weight in Kilograms

		45	48	50	53	55	58	60	63	65	68	70	73	75	78	80	82.5	85	87.5	90
	145.0	21.4	22.6	23.8	25.0	26.2	27.3	28.5	29.7	30.9	32.1	33.3	34.5	35.7	36.9	38.0	39.2	40.4	41.6	42.8
	147.5	20.7	21.8	23.0	24.1	25.3	26.4	27.6	28.7	29.9	31.0	32.2	33.3	34.5	35.6	36.8	37.9	39.1	40.2	41.4
	150.0	20.0	21.1	22.2	23.3	24.4	25.6	26.7	27.8	28.9	30.0	31.1	32.2	33.3	34.4	35.6	36.7	37.8	38.9	40.0
	152.5	19.3	20.4	21.5	22.6	23.6	24.7	25.8	26.9	27.9	29.0	30.1	31.2	32.2	33.3	34.4	35.5	36.5	37.6	38.7
	155.0	18.7	19.8	20.8	21.9	22.9	23.9	25.0	26.0	27.1	28.1	29.1	30.2	31.2	32.3	33.3	34.3	35.4	36.4	37.5
	157.5	18.1	19.1	20.2	21.2	22.2	23.2	24.2	25.2	26.2	27.2	28.2	29.2	30.2	31.2	32.2	33.3	34.3	35.3	36.3
Height in Centimeters	160.0	17.6	18.6	19.5	20.5	21.5	22.5	23.4	24.4	25.4	26.4	27.3	28.3	29.3	30.3	31.3	32.2	33.2	34.2	35.2
	162.5	17.0	18.0	18.9	19.9	20.8	21.8	22.7	23.7	24.6	25.6	26.5	27.5	28.4	29.3	30.3	31.2	32.2	33.1	34.1
	165.0	16.5	17.4	18.4	19.3	20.2	21.1	22.0	23.0	23.9	24.8	25.7	26.6	27.5	28.5	29.4	30.3	31.2	32.1	33.1
	167.5	16.0	16.9	17.8	18.7	19.6	20.5	21.4	22.3	23.2	24.1	24.9	25.8	26.7	27.6	28.5	29.4	30.3	31.2	32.1
	170.0	15.6	16.4	17.3	18.2	19.0	19.9	20.8	21.6	22.5	23.4	24.2	25.1	26.0	26.8	27.7	28.5	29.4	30.3	31.1
	172.5	15.1	16.0	16.8	17.6	18.5	19.3	20.2	21.0	21.8	22.7	23.5	24.4	25.2	26.0	26.9	27.7	28.6	29.4	30.2
	175.0	14.7	15.5	16.3	17.1	18.0	18.8	19.6	20.4	21.2	22.0	22.9	23.7	24.5	25.3	26.1	26.9	27.8	28.6	29.4
	177.5	14.3	15.1	15.9	16.7	17.5	18.3	19.0	19.8	20.6	21.4	22.2	23.0	23.8	24.6	25.4	26.2	27.0	27.8	28.6
	180.0	13.9	14.7	15.4	16.2	17.0	17.7	18.5	19.3	20.1	20.8	21.6	22.4	23.1	23.9	24.7	25.5	26.2	27.0	27.8
	182.5	13.5	14.3	15.0	15.8	16.5	17.3	18.0	18.8	19.5	20.3	21.0	21.8	22.5	23.3	24.0	24.8	25.5	26.3	27.0
	185.0	13.1	13.9	14.6	15.3	16.1	16.8	17.5	18.3	19.0	19.7	20.5	21.2	21.9	22.6	23.4	24.1	24.8	25.6	26.3
	187.5	12.8	13.5	14.2	14.9	15.6	16.4	17.1	17.8	18.5	19.2	19.9	20.6	21.3	22.0	22.8	23.5	24.2	24.9	25.6
	190.0	12.5	13.2	13.9	14.5	15.2	15.9	16.6	17.3	18.0	18.7	19.4	20.1	20.8	21.5	22.2	22.9	23.5	24.2	24.9

http://www.freebmicalculator.net

█ Underweight   █ Normal   █ Overweight   █ Obesity

Figure 5.4 The body mass index calculator.

> " The first time I used the BMI calculator was with the health visitor
> on my second placement so when I was asked to calculate the BMI
> of an elderly frail patient I felt really on top it. It just takes practice
> and confidence. Jade, third year student

When the BMI has been calculated the other steps in the process have to be undertaken. The final step, step 5, guides the nurse with regards to the most appropriate management strategy. The patient's overall risk score must be recorded and an individualised care plan devised. The care plan must be documented so that all health care providers can refer to it. Table 5.3 provides a brief overview of the management to be taken when the MUST score has been determined.

Patients who are in the high- or medium-risk groups will often require some form of intervention. The care plan should describe the aims and objectives of treatment and care interventions and these will be monitored and reviewed. The patient must be reassessed for nutritional risk as they journey through different care settings.

Table 5.3 An overview of the management to be taken when the MUST score has been established

MUST score	Overall risk of malnutrition	Activity
2 or more	High	Treat, unless harmful or no benefit from nutritional support expected, for example if death is imminent
1	Medium	Observe, or treat if the patient is approaching high risk or if sudden and rapid clinical deterioration expected
0	Low	Routine care, unless major clinical decline is expected

In those patients who have been determined to be obese, any underlying acute conditions are usually controlled prior to treating obesity. *Source*: adapted BAPEN (2011).

ACTIVITY 5.5

Go to this page on the BAPEN website (www.bapen.org .uk/pdfs/must/must_explan.pdf) where you will find the MUST booklet, which has a great deal of information about the MUST tool. There are a number of flow charts that will help you understand how all of the steps associated with the tool fit together to enable you to undertake a full assessment of the patient's nutritional needs.

 ## Modified Early Warning Score

Early identification of the risk of clinical deterioration and the ability to escalate concerns have become important activities that all nurses must possess. Most patients admitted to hospital progress and do well and are discharged in good health. There are times, however, when a patient's health status deteriorates and their condition requires further, sometimes intensive intervention.

The Modified Early Warning Score (MEWS) is a type of track-and-trigger scoring system. The triggers used are based on routine observations and are so sensitive that they have the ability to detect any subtle changes in a patient's physiology; this is reflected by a change in score as the patient's condition improves or deteriorates.

Patient vital signs can be converted into a score, and the higher the score then the more abnormal the vital signs are. If the scores reach a predetermined threshold then actions are put in place where a senior nurse/clinician and or a doctor must be called to carry out an assessment of the patient.

The rationale underpinning early warning scoring systems is associated with two specific aims:

1 to facilitate timely recognition of patients with established or impending critical illness,
2 to empower nurses to secure experienced help through the operation of a trigger threshold, which, if reached, requires compulsory attendance by a more senior member of staff.

Using a MEWS can also:

- enhance the quality of patient observation and monitoring,
- improve communication within the multidisciplinary team,
- ensure timely admission to acute assessment units/intensive care,
- support good nursing/medical judgement,
- help in securing appropriate assistance for those patients whose condition is clinically deteriorating,
- provide a good indication of physiological trends,
- be a sensitive indicator of abnormal physiology.

PEARLS OF WISDOM

A MEWS is not:
- a predictor of outcome,
- a comprehensive clinical assessment tool,
- a replacement for clinical judgement.

Track-and-trigger systems have been introduced to reduce the number of adverse incidents that can occur when a patient (who may or may not be acutely ill) deteriorates. It is essential to recognise deterioration and act quickly. In 1998 a confidential inquiry into the quality of care before admission to intensive care considered why patients admitted from a ward area were much less likely to survive intensive care than those coming from an accident and emergency department or the operating theatre (McQuillan et al., 1998). This study determined that:

- 41% of admissions to intensive care may have been avoidable if earlier intervention had occurred,
- 69% of admissions to intensive care occurred late in the development of critical illness,
- 54% of admissions had suboptimal care prior to admission.

The study highlighted the role of an early warning scoring system in the early recognition and management of high-risk patients. The use of MEWS was a significant recommendation of the later National Confidential Enquiry into Patient Outcome and Death (2005) study and report.

The use of MEWS

The use of MEWS as a track-and-trigger system relies on the routine recording and charting of the physiological status of the patient (that is, their observations). These observations can be performed by a nurse and other trained staff, such as healthcare assistants and assistant practitioners.

The National Institute for Health and Care Excellence (NICE, 2007a) has recommended that physiological track-and-trigger scoring systems should be used in monitoring all patients in the acute care setting, with each patient being monitored at least every 12 hours. There are six physiological parameters that NICE (2007a) identified as essential:

- respiratory rate,
- oxygen saturations,
- heart rate,
- systolic blood pressure,
- temperature,
- level of consciousness.

Other physiological measurements (observations) can be included; for example:

- urine output,
- degree of oedema,
- pain score,
- nutritional score,
- score on the Glasgow Coma Scale.

It is usual that all patients will have their observations carried out and a MEWS score charted on admission to the ward. The frequency and specific details of the observations will be described clearly in the nursing care plan.

There are some patients who are considered to be at high risk of developing a critical illness and as such good practice dictates that it would be appropriate to commence the track-and-trigger system at the earliest opportunity. These patients would include (but are not exclusive to) the following:

- all patients admitted as an emergency,
- those patients whose condition is unstable (labile),
- patients whose condition is causing concern,
- patients requiring frequent or an increasing frequency of observations,
- patients who have been stepped down from a higher level of care,
- patients with a chronic health problem,
- patients who are failing to progress as expected.

Although the majority of patients may benefit from the utilisation of a track-and-trigger system the nurse's own clinical judgement will dictate whether or not the person needs to be scored regularly. The decision to use or not to use a track-and-trigger system must be clearly documented, with the rationale for action detailed in the person's care plan.

The MEWS chart

A standard MEWS system is usually used across all directorates and specialties in an acute trust. Community MEWS are an adaptation of the MEWS and are used by nurses caring for the increasing number of acutely ill people in the community setting. The triggers are adapted to meet the needs of the care setting. The MEWS is often incorporated into the standard observation chart (see Figure 5.5).

SCORE...	3	2	1	0	1	2	3
Pulse rate (beats per minute)		<40	41–50	51–90	91–110	111–130	≥131
Respiratory rate (breaths per minute)	< 8		9–11	12–20		21–24	≥25
Temperature (°C)	≤35.0		35.1–36.0	36.1–38.0	38.1–39.0	≥39.1	
Systolic blood pressure (mmHg)	≤90	91–80	81–100	111–249	>250		
Oxygen saturations	<88%	92–93%	94–95%	>96%		Any O$_2$	
AVPU scale				A			V, P, U

Figure 5.5 An aggregate weighted track-and-trigger system. AVPU is a simple assessment where A = alert, V = responds to verbal commands only, P = responds to pain and U = completely unresponsive. *Source:* adapted from Prytherch *et al.* (2010) and Resuscitation Council UK (2011).

PEARLS OF WISDOM

Prior to being allocated to any care area (or at least as you enter the care area) you should always find out the number for the cardiac arrest team and any other emergency numbers/contacts you might need to use should an emergency arise during your placement.

MEWS scores that will trigger action

Trigger scores will be devised locally and it is essential that the nurse is aware of what score determines what intervention. A MEWS score of 2 in any category indicates the need for close and frequent observation of the patient. A MEWS score of 4 and/or an increase of 2 or more indicates that the patient is potentially unwell and that urgent medical attention is required. A MEWS action plan must be agreed and documented for any patient reviewed. It is essential that documentation is clear and contemporaneous.

ACTIVITY 5.6

Calculate the MEWS score for Mr Bhupinder Gujral, aged 63, who was admitted with a 3-day history of a productive cough; he is expectorating copious amounts of green, tenacious sputum. His condition has failed to improve despite the administration of prescribed antibiotics and bronchodilators. Bhupinder is extremely breathless.

- Pulse, 120 beats per minute
- Temperature, 37.6°C
- Respiratory rate, 24 breaths per minute
- Systolic blood pressure, 125 mmHg
- S_pO_2, 93%
- Bhupinder responds to verbal commands only

What action will you take? How will you escalate your concerns to prevent further deterioration? What does the track-and-trigger tool on your ward require that you do when you have calculated the score?

 ## Glasgow Coma Scale

The Glasgow Coma Scale (GCS) is a neurological assessment scale and provides nurses with an objective way of recording the conscious state. The GCS was initially used to assess the level of consciousness after head injury and was published in 1974 by Graham Teasdale and Bryan J. Jennett at the University of Glasgow. It is now used universally (Teasdale and Jennett, 1974).

This assessment tool is made up of three components:

1 best eye-opening response,
2 best verbal response,
3 best motor response.

Within each element there are subcategories and a corresponding score is awarded (see Table 5.4).

Table 5.4. The Glasgow Coma Scale

Best eye-opening response (record 1(C) if unable to open eyes, e.g. from orbital swelling or facial fractures)	Eyes open spontaneously	4
	Eyes open to speech	3
	Eyes open to pain	2
	No eye opening	1
Best verbal response (record 1(T) if the person has a endotracheal or tracheostomy tube in place and record 1(D) if the person is dysphasic)	Orientated to time and place	5
	Confused	4
	Inappropriate words	3
	Incomprehensible sounds	2
	No verbal response	1
Best motor response	Obeys commands	6
	Localises to pain	5
	Withdrawal from pain	4
	Flexion to pain	3
	Extension to pain	2
	No motor response	1

Source: Teasdale and Jennett (1974).

Altered consciousness consists of abnormal behaviour in one or more of the three functional areas in Table 5.4. The maximum score a patient can score is 15/15 and the worst possible score is 3/15. There are some patients who may be unable to speak as a result of therapeutic interventions, for example they may have been intubated or have a tracheostomy tube in situ, and in these instances the patient is unable to respond verbally as they have no air passing over the vocal cords. If this situation arises the nurse scores the patient a verbal score of 1 and marks 1(T) on the chart: this indicates that intubation is causing the verbal deficit. It is the same for those patients who are unable to open the eyes due to swelling or orbital fracture, which is recorded as 1(C). In most patients a GCS score of 8 or less would indicate unconsciousness.

Although the GCS is meant to be an objective assessment of the patient's level of consciousness, there is a degree of subjectivity associated with it. The nurse assessing the patient's GCS makes a judgement concerning the responses the patient makes to stimuli and as such it is inevitable that there will be a degree of subjectivity. For this element of subjectivity to be reduced it is suggested that where possible nurses assess the GCS jointly. NICE (2007b) suggests that if the GCS deteriorates then a second competent nurse should immediately check the GCS, confirming the deterioration before informing or seeking assistance from the medical team.

Hickey (2009) suggests that level of consciousness is the most important feature of the neurological assessment. Level of consciousness is the earliest and most sensitive indicator of neurological deterioration.

Using the GCS to assess a patient's neurological status requires much skill and as you become more familiar with it your confidence will grow (as is the case with all of the assessment tools discussed in this chapter). The AVPU scale (referred to in the MEWS discussion) can give information easily and quickly about the person's level of consciousness. However, in those patients with neurological conditions the AVPU is an inadequate assessment tool and should not be used as an alternative to the GCS (see Table 5.5).

Table 5.5 The AVPU scale

A = alert	Is the person alert?
V = responds to voice	Do they respond to verbal stimulation?
P = responds to pain	Do they respond to pain?
U = unresponsive	Do they respond at all?

Best motor response is the next aspect to be assessed: Table 5.4 shows that there are six possible responses the patient could make, and so the motor response section of the GCS carries the most weight. Repeated practice and watching more senior experienced nurses will make you much more adept at assessing best motor response.

 Assessing motor response is really complicated. I was working with a senior staff nurse who had to apply painful stimuli to assess the patient's response. The patient was unconscious, it seemed so cruel, but it was the only way to obtain a true assessment of the patient's needs. We explained all of this to the patient's family. *Karolina, second year student*

Assessing muscle strength in the conscious and unconscious patient requires different approaches. A scale to grade muscle strength is used to allocate scores to the strength of muscle (see Table 5.6).

Table 5.6 Grading of muscle strength

Grade	Indicator of limb power
5	Active movement against gravity, full resistance, normal strength
4	Active movement against gravity, some resistance that can be overcome by the examiner
3	Active movement against gravity, unable to resist the examiner
2	Active movement when gravity is eliminated
1	No active movement, weak muscle contraction can be palpated
0	No muscle contraction detected

Assessing pupil size and reaction

Making an assessment of the way the pupils react (or not) to light and assessing the character of the pupils is not part of the scoring system of the GCS, but is an essential component of neurological assessment. Undertaking this assessment can assist in identifying the location of a potentially expanding space-occupying lesion and is also a later sign of raised intracranial pressure. If you notice any changes in pupil reaction, shape or size this should be reported and documented immediately.

Pupil size, pupil shape, reactivity to light and equality of pupil size should be assessed and recorded on the neurological observation chart. If they are unable to be assessed due to oedema a C should be entered on the chart. A plus sign (+) indicates pupil reactivity on the neurological observation chart, and a minus sign (−) indicates no reaction.

PEARLS OF WISDOM

- Seventeen per cent of the normal population have unequal pupil sizes, known as anisocoria.
- Be aware that some medication may influence the size of the pupil.
- Pre-existing ophthalmic conditions can produce a unilaterally dilated pupil; for example, cataract or localised injury, or misshapen pupils in people who have undergone cataract surgery.
- Those patients who have prosthetic eyes will not show a reaction to light in that eye.

 Summary

The nursing process uses a systematic, holistic, problem-solving approach in partnership with the patient and their family. Assessment is the first stage in the nursing process. Nurses use every tool available to gather the information required to compile a patient's diagnoses and to formulate a care plan.

There are a number of assessment tools available to nurses to help them undertake an objective assessment of the needs of patients. Assessment tools are designed to encapsulate a systematic approach to assessment while at the same time incorporating professional decision making that takes place between a nurse and the patient. When using an assessment tool the nurse should work through a staged approach, moving from the general to the specific, focusing assessment activity on aspects of risk and complexity.

It is important to note that assessment tools are not designed to replace the nurses' clinical judgement. The assessment domains within the tool should act as triggers for specialist assessment.

Developing the appropriate skills to undertake a safe and effective assessment of needs takes time and commitment. As the nurse develops, observes skilled nurses at work and practices under supervision, confidence and competence will grow.

 # References

British Association for Parenteral and Enteral Nutrition (2011) *The 'MUST' Explanatory Book-let.* www.bapen.org.uk/pdfs/must/must_explan.pdf

Burke, K.M., Mohn-Brown, E.L. and Eby, L. (2011) *Medical-Surgical Nursing Care*, 3rd edn. Pearson, Boston

Griffiths, P. (2009) Top nurse warns risk assessment tools are not backed evidence. *Nursing Times* 8 Dec

Hickey, J. V. (2009) *Clinical Practice of Neurological & Neurosurgical Nursing*, 6th edn. Lippincott Williams and Wilkins, Philadelphia

McQuillan, P., Pilkington, S., Allan, A., Taylor, B., Short, A., Morgan, G., Nielson, M., Barrett, D. and Smith, G. (1998) Confidential enquiry into quality of care before admission to intensive care. *British Medical Journal* 316, 1853–8

National Confidential Enquiry into Patient Outcome and Death (2005) *An Acute Problem?* National Confidential Enquiry into Patient Outcome and Death, London

NICE (2007a) *Head Injury: Triage, Assessment, Investigation and Early Management of Head Injury in Infants, Children and Adults*. Clinical Guideline 56. http://publications.nice.org.uk/head-injury-cg56

NICE (2007b) *Acutely Ill Patients in Hospital*. Clinical Guideline 50. National Institute for Health and Clinical Excellence, London

Prytherch, D., Smith, G., Schmidt, P. and Featherstone, P. (2010) ViEWS – towards a national Early Warning Score for detecting inpatient deterioration. *Resuscitation* 81(8), 932–7

Resuscitation Council UK (2011) *Immediate Life Support*, 3rd edn. Resuscitation Council, UK

Teasdale, G. and Jennett, B.J. (1974) Assessment of coma and impaired consciousness. A practical scale. *Lancet* 2(7872), 81–4

Yara, H. and Walsh, M. (1967) *The Nursing Process*. Appleton-Century-Crofts, Norwalk, CT

 # Resources

British Association for Parenteral and Enteral Nutrition
www.bapen.org.uk/
BAPEN exists to help ensure that those suffering from malnutrition or other nutritional problems are appropriately recognised and managed. The organisation encourages the development of an integrated approach to managed nutritional care, improving the nutritional care of people at risk of malnutrition in hospitals or in the community.

Guidelines and Audit Implementation Network
www.gain-ni.org/
GAIN is associated with audit, guidelines, teaching and medical device evaluation shaped by all staff in health and social care in Northern Ireland, with the single aim of benefiting patients and championing quality and best practice.

National Institute for Health and Clinical Excellence
www.nice.org.uk/
NICE guidance supports healthcare professionals and others to ensure that the care they offer is of the best possible quality and is the best value for money.

Resuscitation Council UK

www.resus.org.uk/

The Resuscitation Council UK provides education and reference materials to healthcare professionals and the general public in the most effective methods of resuscitation.

Scottish Intercollegiate Guidelines Network

www.sign.ac.uk/

The Scottish Intercollegiate Guidelines Network (SIGN) develops evidence-based clinical practice guidelines for the NHS in Scotland. SIGN guidelines are derived from a systematic review of the scientific literature and are designed as a vehicle for accelerating the translation of new knowledge into action to reduce variations in practice and improving patient outcomes.

CHAPTER 6

The Essential Skills Clusters

WHAT THIS CHAPTER CONTAINS

- The NHS Constitution
- A discussion of the rationale for essential skills clusters
- Care, compassion and communication
- Organisational aspects of care
- Infection, prevention and control
- Nutrition and fluid management
- Medicines management
- Numerical skills assessment

The NHS Constitution

The NHS Constitution (Department of Health, 2012) has been produced to protect and renew the principles of the NHS. It has the ability to empower staff, patients and the public by describing existing legal rights and assurances for the first time in one place. Although the core principles of the NHS are shared across all four countries of the UK the NHS Constitution applies only to the NHS in England. The devolved administrations in Scotland, Wales and Northern Ireland are responsible for developing their own health policies.

NHS values, expressed in the NHS Constitution provide common ground for cooperation to achieve shared aspirations. Every nurse should aspire to meet and exceed the values and principles listed below.

Respect and dignity: nurses value each person as an individual, respect their ambitions and commitments in life and aim to understand their priorities, needs, abilities and limits.

Commitment to quality of care: as nurses we earn the trust placed in us by insisting on quality and endeavouring to get the fundamentals right every time with specific emphasis on safety, confidentiality, professional integrity, accountability, dependable service and effective communication. We value feedback, learn from our mistakes and build on our successes.

The Student Nurse Toolkit: An Essential Guide for Surviving Your Course, First Edition. Ian Peate.
© 2013 John Wiley & Sons, Ltd. Published 2013 by John Wiley & Sons, Ltd.

Compassion: we respond with humanity and kindness to each person's pain, distress, anxiety or need. We do things, no matter how small, to offer comfort and alleviate suffering. We find time for those we serve and we work alongside them. Because we care we do not wait to be asked.

Improving lives: it is our endeavour to work with people to improve health and well-being and people's experiences of the services we offer. We value excellence and professionalism in the things that enhance people's lives in nursing care, clinical practice, service improvements and innovation.

Working together for patients: patients are our first concern in everything we do, working in partnership with other staff, patients, carers, families, communities and a wide range of other professionals. The needs of the people we serve transcend organisational boundaries.

Everyone counts: the work nurses do and the resources available are there for the benefit of the whole community. We endeavour to ensure that nobody is excluded or left behind. We acknowledge that some people will need more help than others, that difficult decisions have to be taken and that the resources available will have to be put to the best use to benefit people and communities. As nurses we are aware that we all have a part to play in making ourselves and our communities healthier.

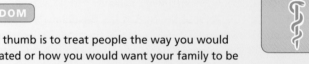

PEARLS OF WISDOM

A good rule of thumb is to treat people the way you would want to be treated or how you would want your family to be treated, but always acknowledge and respect the fact that we are all individual, we are all different.

The essential skills clusters

The essential skills clusters (ESCs) were introduced into the pre-registration nursing curriculum in 2007 (Nursing and Midwifery Council, 2007a) and they are still an integral element of the revised 2010 pre-registration standards (Nursing and Midwifery Council, 2010a). Every nursing student in the UK must be able to demonstrate competence to meet the criteria for registration with the NMC. The NMC has determined that the ESCs are to be used as guidance and must be incorporated into all pre-registration nursing programmes. How the ESCs are incorporated into programmes of study is left to local determination, so each university may have a different approach to the teaching and assessment of competence associated with the ESCs.

The ESC learning outcomes can be developed at different levels and they apply to the four fields of nursing. See Box 6.1 for the five ESCs.

Box 6.1 The five ESCs

1 Care, compassion and communication
2 Organisational aspects of care
3 Infection prevention and control
4 Nutrition and fluid management
5 Medicines management

Each ESC begins with a statement of achievement explaining the skills and behaviours that the newly qualified graduate nurse should be able to demonstrate prior to being allowed entry to the professional register. The NMC code of conduct (the *Code*; Nursing and Midwifery Council, 2008) and *Guidance on Professional Conduct for Nursing and Midwifery Students* (Nursing and Midwifery Council, 2010b) have been used to focus the ESCs and as such features of those documents are found in the ESC outcomes.

ACTIVITY 6.1

Make a comparison of the NMC *Code* (Nursing and Midwifery Council, 2008) and the *Guidance on Professional Conduct for Nursing and Midwifery Students* (Nursing and Midwifery Council, 2010b). Look at how the content of both important documents underpin the content of the ESCs.

There are also elements of the NHS Constitution (Department of Health, 2012) intertwined in the ESCs.

Many of the standards expected of the student nurse in the ESCs will assume that you will be able to engender trust in the public and the people you have the privilege to serve. You should always remember that some of the people you offer care to will often be at a stage in their lives when they are at their most vulnerable: they may be in pain, they may be scared, and they will look to you to offer them kindness and compassion. You can only do this through open, effective communication.

All of the ESCs described here have an element of trust associated with them as well as what it is that the public should expect from a newly qualified graduate nurse.

> For each placement I go to, I take with me my list of skills that I am to be assessed on. It really helps me and my mentor to focus on what it is that needs to be achieved. I used to be so keen (sometimes too keen) to get them all done as soon as possible, but now I think, take it easy, you've lots of time to do this.
> *Christopher, first year student*

One of the fundamental elements of good nursing is good communication with patients. Failure to communicate effectively with a patient when we first meet them can destroy the intricate nurse–patient relationship and lead to the patient not trusting the nurse.

Care, compassion and communication

There are eight components associated with care, compassion and communication. It is expected the person being cared for can trust the newly qualified graduate nurse to:

1 work in partnership to provide collaborative care based on the highest standards, knowledge and competence,
2 engage in person-centred care, empowering people to make choices about how their needs are to be met,
3 respect people as individuals, helping them to preserve their dignity at all times,
4 engage with the people cared for and their family or carers within their cultural environments in an acceptant and anti-discriminatory manner,
5 provide care that is delivered in a warm, sensitive and compassionate way,
6 engage with people therapeutically and to actively listen to their needs and concerns, using skills that are helpful, providing information that is clear, accurate, meaningful and free from jargon,
7 maintain confidentiality,
8 gain informed consent prior to any intervention.

It is easy to communicate but, to communicate effectively is much more difficult. Being an effective communicator requires much skill. A great deal has been written on communication and maybe this is because we often fail to communicate effectively with each other, with other healthcare professionals and with the people for whom we care and their families.

The NHS Constitution (Department of Health, 2012) highlights the importance of good communication with the aim of building trust between healthcare providers and patients and their families. Poor communication is still one of the most common reasons why people make complaints about the NHS. Poor communication while delivering care or treatment can be made worse when nurses fail to listen and respond sensitively; the outcome of this can be an overall care experience that leaves a patient or their family feeling that they have not been listened to or that their individual needs have been neglected. Nurses and other healthcare professionals failing to communicate effectively can damage successful clinical treatment, resulting in a patient's story of their experience with healthcare providers changing from one of success to one that leaves them feeling frustrated, anxious and dissatisfied.

In February 2011 the Parliamentary and Health Service Ombudsman (2011) published a report called *Care and Compassion?* This report described the Ombudsman's findings in relation to 10 investigations into NHS care of older people. The report revealed the unnecessary pain, indignity and distress being experienced by older people in hospital or under the care of their GP. It was revealed that there was a gap between the principles and values of the NHS Constitution and the poor quality of care experienced by the patients whose cases were investigated.

The report *Care and Compassion?* concluded that the NHS was failing to meet even the most basic standards of care as a result of attitudes – both personal and institutional – that did not recognise the humanity and individuality of older people and failed to respond to them with sensitivity, compassion and professionalism.

Communication is at the heart of any relationship, be it familial, professional, romantic or friendship. Communication can be described as a process of exchanging information, ideas, thoughts, feelings and emotions through speech, signals, writing or behaviour (Almond and Yardley, 2009). The process of communication requires a sender (encoder) who encodes a message and then uses a medium/channel to send it to the receiver (decoder) who decodes the message. After processing information the decoder sends back appropriate feedback/reply using a medium/channel (see Figure 6.1); these are the components of effective communication.

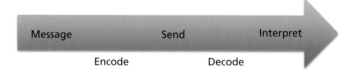

Figure 6.1 The communication process.

When nurses communicate effectively with patients and their families they will be able to ensure that the care they are providing is kind, compassionate and respectful, because they are listening to and acting in the patient's best interests.

PEARLS OF WISDOM

Effective nursing communication is about getting the right information to the right person in the right format at the right time in the right location, all done in such a way that is easily understandable.

Types of communication

There are various types of communication and the method chosen often depends on the message and the context in which it is being sent. The chosen communication channel and the style of communicating can also affect communication. Verbal communication is one of the most important aspects of how we interact with other people.

Verbal communication

Verbal communication has a number of advantages over other forms of communication; for example, when we speak we can slow down and present points one by one. As we continue we can ensure that each point is clear and has been understood before moving to the next point. This can have the potential to increase the accuracy of communication.

Verbal communication can be much more precise than when we use nonverbal cues. Verbal communication is enhanced when it is combined with other forms of communication such as body language and gestures.

There are also disadvantages associated with verbal communication and there are times when verbal communication is not the best option. When we use verbal communication there is a reduced chance of an objective record of the interaction being made, and the spoken word can also be forgotten quickly, especially if there are multiple points to consider, so recall may be problematic. As with all types of communication there is always the risk of miscommunication leading to inappropriate responses.

Nonverbal communication

This type of communication is any kind of communication that does not involve the use of words. Nonverbal communication can include more than just facial expressions and gestures it also includes vocal sounds that are not words; for example, grunts, sighs and whimpers. Even when we use actual words, there are nonverbal sound elements such as voice tone, pacing of speech and so forth.

The way we dress can also provide others with nonverbal communication. When nurses wear a uniform they are communicating an important message even before a word has been said: the uniform acts as a cue. Cues convey messages, and so too does their absence. In some settings failing to express a nonverbal cue communicates meaning. A nurse who fails to adhere to the uniform policy, or who looks slovenly or unkempt, is conveying a very different message to the nurse who wears a uniform as dictated by policy; some would consider the former less professional. Dressing down in this case implies a relaxation of professional standards that entails much more than just a change of clothes.

There are also some nonverbal cues that are based on learned cultural standards, but there are some elements of nonverbal communication that are universal, such as anger, fear, sadness and surprise.

The setting where communication occurs also contributes to the meaning of words besides their literal definition, and this also constitutes nonverbal communication. For instance, the sign of a cross has much cultural meaning when used in a religious context, yet when it is seen on a road sign it means merely that there is a junction ahead.

Some types of nonverbal communication that accompany words are known as modifiers, which alter meanings. For example, the speed of our speech and the pauses we put between the spoken words form a nonverbal element to our speech, and they modify it. A slight pause or hesitation before a word may suggest uncertainty, or can be interpreted as a request for the listener to confirm something. However, when there are no pauses it implies that the speaker is confident about what they are saying. If you are asked a question in a hurried way, it may feel that the person is expecting you to make a quick reply.

ACTIVITY 6.2

List five emotions that you think you have shown in the last week. With a friend talk about how you were able to identify what those emotions were. Once you have discussed several emotions, act some emotions out with a friend. Have your friend try to guess which emotion you are representing. Swap places and have your friend act out some.

Think about emotions that sometimes look the same. What parts of the body do you look at when you are trying to understand a person's emotions? Do you feel that many emotions have actions that are clearly recognisable?

Another form of nonverbal communication is the use of personal space. By leaning towards their listener as they speak, a person may infer that they are communicating something that is personal or a secret. Subject to the social nuances of the situation, this could be taken as a sign of friendship or even an unwanted invasion of space.

Haptic communication is to do with the use of touching when used as an element of communication; the meanings associated with touch are very culture-dependent. In some societies a handshake is an acceptable means of greeting a person, in others this may be unacceptable and can be seen as an invasion of personal space.

The use of the eyes, occulesics, when used as an aspect of nonverbal communication is an important element of nonverbal communication. Eye movements can be divided into separate elements; for example, the number and length of eye contacts, how many times the person blinks and pupil dilation. The cues and the interpretation of these cues are dependent on the culture of the participants. A protracted stare can result in the establishment of a bond of trust, or could just as easily destroy it.

Nonverbal communication is how most of our communication occurs. When we compare the verbal and nonverbal communication that happens between us, it is the nonverbal part that is by far the greatest aspect of how we convey our message (see Figure 6.2).

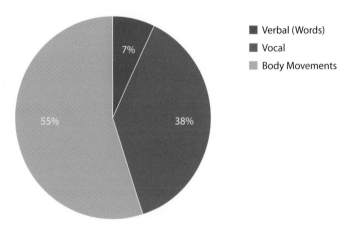

Figure 6.2 Breakdown of verbal and nonverbal communication.

> *We did an exercise at uni in year one where we had to record a mock-up of a patient–nurse interaction and we got to keep the CD. I still have that CD and I cringe when I see how my nonverbals were loaded with negatives, my eye movement – rolling my eyes to the sky, I learned loads from this. Janet, third year student*

Maintaining confidentiality

Nurses have a professional and legal duty to maintain confidentiality. The NMC code of professional conduct (Nursing and Midwifery Council, 2008) states that nurses must:

- respect people's right to confidentiality,
- ensure people are informed about how and why information is shared by those who will be providing their care,

🔖 disclose information if you believe someone may be at risk of harm, in line with the law of the country in which you are practising.

A duty of confidence comes about when one person discloses information to another in situations where it is reasonable to expect that the information will be kept in confidence (Nursing and Midwifery Council, 2009). This duty of confidence is derived from common law (the decisions of the Courts) and statute law which is passed by Parliament.

Confidentiality is an essential aspect of professional practice that respects human rights. Article 8 (Right to respect for private and family life) of the European Convention of Human Rights refers to confidentiality.

Under common law people have a right to expect that information given to a nurse be only used for the purpose for which it was given and that this will not be disclosed without permission. This also applies to situations where information is disclosed directly to the nurse and also to information that the nurse obtains from others.

One element of privacy is that individuals have the right to control access to their own personal health information. It is unacceptable to:

🔖 discuss matters related to the people in your care outside the clinical setting,
🔖 discuss a case with colleagues when you are in public and where you may be overheard,
🔖 leave records unattended where they may be read by unauthorised persons (this is discussed further in Chapter 15 of this book).

 Disclosure

There are instances when you may need to disclose information given to you. Disclosure is only lawful and ethical if the individual has given their consent for that information to be passed on, such consent must be freely and fully given. Consent to disclosure of confidential information may be:

🔖 explicit,
🔖 implied,
🔖 required by law, or
🔖 capable of justification by reason of the public interest.

 Disclosure with consent

Explicit consent is obtained when the person you are caring for agrees to disclosure having been informed of the reason for that disclosure and with whom the information may or will be shared. Explicit consent may be written or spoken.

Implied consent is obtained when it is assumed that the person being cared for understands that their information may be shared within the healthcare team. You are required to make the people in your care aware of this routine sharing of information; if there are any objections you should record these clearly.

Disclosure without consent

The term 'public interest' describes the exceptional circumstances that validate overruling the right of an individual to confidentiality with the intention of serving a broader social concern.

Staff are permitted under common law to disclose personal information in order to prevent and support detection, investigation and punishment of a serious crime and/or to prevent abuse or serious harm to others. It is important that each case be judged on its merits. The Nursing and Midwifery Council (2009) suggests the following examples could include disclosing information in relation to crimes against the person:

- ☥ rape,
- ☥ child abuse,
- ☥ murder,
- ☥ kidnapping,
- ☥ a result of injuries sustained from knife or gunshot wounds.

These are complex decisions and they must take account both the public interest in ensuring confidentiality and the public interest in disclosure. Advice from a senior manager should be sought prior to disclosing any information.

Disclosure to third parties

Where information is shared with other people and/or organisations not directly involved in a person's care this is deemed disclosure to a third party. Nurses must ensure that those people in their care are made aware that information about them could be disclosed to third parties involved in their care. The patient may object to the use and disclosure of confidential information and if this is the case it should be clearly documented.

The Department of Health (2003) has produced an *NHS Code of Practice* related to confidentiality; there is also supplementary guidance available regarding public interests disclosure (Department of Health, 2010). Both publications are underpinned by the Data Protection Act 1988. Further discussion concerning the law and consent can be found in Chapter 16.

SECTION SUMMARY

Failure to communicate effectively can have a detrimental effect on the care delivered. Effective communication means that the nurse has to understand the principles underpinning communication. Accepting a person unconditionally, without judging them in a genuine way with empathy and positive regard (Rogers, 1957, 1959) demonstrates your commitment to the person being cared for.

Confidentiality is the cornerstone of nursing. People you care for should be able to expect that the information they give you would be kept confidential and shared only with their consent to help with the care they are given or are to receive. There are times when disclosure is required, but these instances are few and far between. If you are required to disclose any information you must seek advice from a senior colleague prior to doing so.

 It's not easy not to judge people, some people do the strangest things, it is not up to me to judge the way people live their lives, but honestly, it's not easy. *Lloyd, third year student*

Organisational aspects of care

There are 12 elements associated with this skills cluster; people should be able to trust the newly registered graduate nurse to:

1 treat people as partners working with them to make a holistic and systematic assessment developing a personalised plan of care,
2 deliver nursing interventions and evaluate effectiveness,
3 safeguard children and adults, support and protect them from harm,
4 respond to feedback, and learn, develop and improve services,
5 promote continuity when care is to be transferred to another service or person,
6 be an autonomous and confident member of the multidisciplinary team,
7 delegate safely to others,
8 lead, co-ordinate and manage care safely,
9 work safely under pressure and maintain the safety of service users,
10 enhance the safety of service users, and identify and actively manage risk,
11 work to prevent and resolve conflict and maintain a safe environment,
12 select and manage medical devices safely.

Previous chapters have discussed the key issues surrounding the provision of individualised care, care planning and the use of a systematic approach to care delivery. A number of assessment tools have already been discussed (see Chapter 5). Understanding and using these will help you, working with the patient and others to identify risk, implementing actions and preventing deterioration in the health and well-being of the people to whom you offer care. Understanding and developing your knowledge base will help to ensure that when you reach the end of your programme (or at other progression points) you will be able to demonstrate competence associated with this ESC.

Infection prevention and control

There are six elements aligned to the infection prevention and control ESC. People should be able to trust the newly registered graduate nurse to:

1 identify and take effective measures to prevent and control infection,
2 maintain effective standards of infection control precautions,
3 provide effective nursing interventions and use standard isolation techniques with people who are infectious,
4 fully comply with hygiene, uniform and dress codes,
5 safely apply with confidence the principles of asepsis when performing invasive procedures,
6 act in a variety of environments, to reduce risk when handling waste, including sharps, contaminated linen and when dealing with spillages of body fluids.

All infection control and prevention activities must be undertaken using a sound evidence base as well as in accordance with local and national policy. The Department of Health (2006) makes it clear that infection control and prevention is the responsibility of everyone.

Pratt *et al.* (2001, 2007) produced national evidence-based guidelines that help to prevent healthcare-associated infections. The guidelines were produced in response to a need to improve patient care and provide robust arrangements for the control and prevention of infection. It is accepted that not all healthcare-associated infection is avoidable, but that nevertheless a significant proportion is preventable. In order to reduce its incidence it was felt that better application of existing knowledge and adherence to good practice would make a major contribution to infection control and prevention; hence the production of the guidelines.

The guidelines are for multiprofessional use, developed following a systematic and expert review of all the available scientific evidence. They cover a number of elements of clinical practice that are an essential part of activity to be taken to prevent the spread of healthcare-associated infection, including multidrug-resistant organisms. Patients with invasive devices such as urinary catheters and peripheral and central venous catheters often require them for life-saving support and treatment. These devices and the fact that they are invasive may also mean that the patient is susceptible to contracting a healthcare-associated infection. One element of best practice is to ensure that you use effective hand-washing hygiene techniques with the intention of reducing the risk of healthcare-associated infection (Kilpatrick *et al.*, 2012). Figure 6.3 provides a diagrammatic representation of the correct procedure required for washing your hands using soap and water.

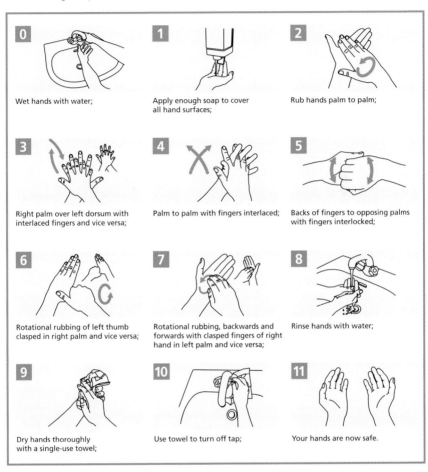

Figure 6.3 How to wash your hands using soap and water. *Source*: World Health Organization (2009).

SECTION SUMMARY

All of us are responsible for ensuring infection prevention and control, no matter where we work. Infection prevention and control is associated with patient safety. The basic skill of hand-washing can have a massive impact on the reduction of healthcare-associated infections.

Nutrition and fluid management

The nutrition and fluid management skills cluster also has six components; people should be able to trust the newly registered graduate nurse to:

1 assist them to choose a diet that provides an adequate nutritional and fluid intake,
2 assess and monitor nutritional status and in partnership, formulate an effective plan of care,
3 assess and monitor fluid status and in partnership with them, formulate an effective plan of care,
4 assist in creating an environment that is conducive to eating and drinking,
5 ensure that those unable to take food by mouth receive adequate fluid and nutrition,
6 safely administer fluids when fluids cannot be taken independently.

In Chapter 5, the Malnutrition Universal Screening Tool (MUST) was described and you were encouraged to become familiar with this tool to be able to demonstrate competence associated with the assessment, planning, implementation and evaluation of care associated with nutrition. This ESC concerns not only nutrition but also fluid management.

The theory underpinning nutrition and fluid management is important but so too are the practical elements associated with this ESC. You need to be able show that you can work with patients and others with the intention of ensuring that the people you care for are receiving adequate and appropriate nutrition and fluids. There are a number of practical skills that you have to learn and become confident with in order to be able to demonstrate competence.

SECTION SUMMARY

As well as understanding the theory underpinning this ESC you must also demonstrate your competence when working with people who require support with their nutritional and fluid needs. You must to be able to assess, plan, implement and evaluate care associated with this ESC.

 Medicines management

The final skills cluster has 10 attributes and again the people you care for should be able to trust you, as a newly registered graduate nurse, to:

1 correctly and safely undertake medicines calculations,
2 work within legal and ethical frameworks,

3 work as part of a team offering holistic care and a range of treatment options of which medicines may form a part,

4 ensure safe and effective practice in medicines management,

5 safely order, receive, store and dispose of medicines (including controlled drugs),

6 administer medicines safely and in a timely manner,

7 keep and maintain accurate records using information technology, where appropriate,

8 work in partnership with people receiving medical treatments and their carers,

9 use and evaluate up-to-date information on medicines management,

10 demonstrate understanding and knowledge to supply and administer via a patient group direction.

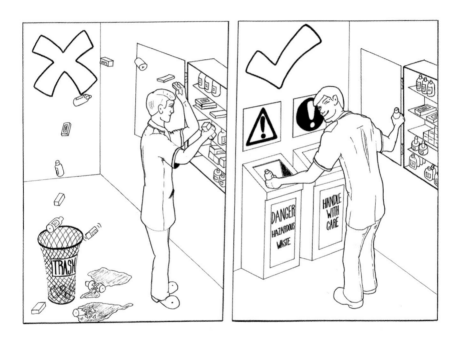

The nurse has a key role to play with respect to the management of medicines. This ESC requires you to be able to demonstrate competence associated with all elements of medicine management including ordering, administering and disposing of medicines.

The NMC has produced detailed standards for medicines management (Nursing and Midwifery Council, 2007b), which you can access on the Internet. Spend some time looking at these detailed standards. The ESC requires you to demonstrate competence in numeracy and drug calculations (see below) and to administer medicines safely via appropriate routes including specific requirements for children and other groups. You need to become conversant with the various routes of administration; for example, intramuscular, subcutaneous, oral, sublingual, pessary and suppository.

You are also required to demonstrate an understanding of the legal and ethical frameworks relating to safe administration of medicines in practice. Chapter 16 provides an overview of the law associated with medicines management.

PEARLS OF WISDOM

When you have some down time, and the pace of work has slowed a little, sit with your mentor and do some drug calculations. Take your time and ask for feedback. Try doing the calculations with and without a calculator.

SECTION SUMMARY

Medicines management incorporates a number of interrelated factors, for example, an understanding of pharmacokinetics, individual choice, numerical assessment, risk management, partnership working and understanding of the law and ethics.

 ## Numerical assessment

Some ESCs require you to use numeracy to calculate medicines, nutritional needs, fluid requirements and other instances where numbers are involved. Universities are required by the NMC to incorporate all these health-related numerical assessments, designed to test numeracy skills, into their learning outcomes and various assessment strategies.

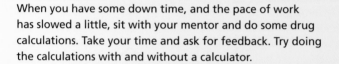

PEARLS OF WISDOM

If you are ever unsure about a calculation that you have made or a colleague has made then question it, seek clarification and refuse to administer any medicine that you think has been incorrectly calculated. Always ask for a second opinion if you doubt yourself or others.

The aim is to be able to demonstrate competence and confidence concerning judgements on whether to use calculations in a particular situation and, if this is the case, what calculations are to be used, how to do them, what degree of accuracy is applicable and how the answer relates to the context of care.

There are many ways in which universities incorporate these health-related numerical elements into learning outcomes and assessment strategies. ESCs should be used to underpin the nature and content of the assessment, and this may include the use of simulation. Assessment can take place in an assortment of settings, ranging from a computer lab to simulated practice (for example, the objective structured clinical examination). However, whatever mode of assessment is chosen it must include assessment in the practice setting.

ACTIVITY 6.3

How many grams in 2 kilograms?

Convert 2.4 L to mL.

Calculate 2.54 m × 2.68 m.

What is 26% of 54?

 ## Summary

The ESCs have been developed to ensure that people can trust the newly registered graduate nurse to demonstrate competence in five key areas. The ESCs form an important part of the assessment process that validates your competence. You will be judged throughout your programme of study in relation to the five ESCs.

This chapter has described the ESCs and their component parts as outlined by the NMC (2007a). The care, compassion and communication ESC was discussed in detail as a failure to demonstrate competence associated with this ESC will also mean that you have not demonstrated competence in the remaining ESCs.

References

Almond, P. and Yardley, J. (2009) An introduction to communication. In Childs, L.L., Coles, L. and Marjoram, B. (eds), *Essential Skills Clusters for Nurses. Theory for Practice*. Wiley, Chichester, pp. 3–17

Department of Health (2003) *Confidentiality: NHS Code of Practice*. Department of Health, London

Department of Health (2006) *The Health Act 2006. Code of Practice for the Prevention and Control of Health Care Associated Infections*. Department of Health, London

Department of Health (2010) *Confidentiality: NHS Code of Practice Supplementary Guidance: Public Interest Disclosure*. Department of Health, London

Department of Health (2012) *The NHS Constitution. The NHS Belongs to us All*. Department of Health, London

Kilpatrick, C., Murdoch, H. and Storr, J. (2012) Importance of hand hygiene during invasive procedures. *Nursing Standard* 26(41), 42–6

Nursing and Midwifery Council (2007a) *Introduction of Essential Skills Clusters for Pre-registration Nursing Programmes*. NMC Circular 07/2007. Nursing and Midwifery Council, London

Nursing and Midwifery Council (2007b) *Standards for Medicines Management*. www.nmc-uk.org/Documents/Standards/nmcStandardsForMedicinesManagementBooklet.pdf

Nursing and Midwifery Council (2008) *The Code: Standards of Conduct, Performance and Ethics for Nurses and Midwives*. Nursing and Midwifery Council, London

Nursing and Midwifery Council (2009) *Advice Sheet: Confidentiality*. www.nmc-uk.org/Nurses-and-midwives/Advice-by-topic/A/Advice/Confidentiality/

Nursing and Midwifery Council (2010a) *Standards for Pre Registration Nursing Education*. http://standards.nmc-uk.org/PublishedDocuments/Standards%20for%20pre-registration%20nursing%20education%2016082010.pdf

Nursing and Midwifery Council (2010b) *Guidance on Professional Conduct for Nursing and Midwifery Students*, 2nd edn. Nursing and Midwifery Council, London

Parliamentary and Health Service Ombudsman (2011) *Care and Compassion?: Report of the Health Service Ombudsman on Ten Investigations into NHS Care of Older People*. TSO, London

Pratt, R., Pellowe, C.M., Wilson, J.A., Loveday, H.P., Robinson, N., Smith, G.W. and the Epic Guideline Development Team (2001) Epic Project: National Evidence-Based Guidelines for Preventing Health Associated Infections. Phase 1. *Journal of Hospital Infection* 47(suppl.), S3–82

Pratt, R., Pellowe, C.M., Wilson, J.A., Loveday, H.P., Harper, P.J., Jones, S.R.L.J., McDougall, C. and Wilcox, M.H. (2007) Epic2: National Evidence-Based Guidelines for Preventing Health Associated Infections in NHS Hospitals in England. *Journal of Hospital Infection* 65(suppl. 1), S1–59

Rogers, C.R. (1957) The necessary and sufficient conditions of therapeutic personality change. *Journal of Consulting Psychology* 21, 95–103

Rogers, C.R. (1959) *A Theory of Therapy, Personality, and Interpersonal Relationships as Developed in the Client-centered Framework*. Reprinted in Kirschenbaum, H. and Henderson, V. (eds) (1989) *The Carl Rogers Reader*. Houghton Mifflin, Boston

World Health Organization (2009) *WHO Guidelines of Hand Hygiene in Health Care*. World Health Organization, Geneva

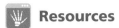 **Resources**

Age UK

www.ageuk.org.uk/

The Age UK Group works to improve later life for everyone by providing life-enhancing services and vital support. It has a vision of a world in which older people flourish, aiming to improve later life for everyone through information and advice, campaigns, products, training and research.

NHS Commissioning Board

www.commissioningboard.nhs.uk/

The NHS Commissioning Board is a Special Health Authority (NHS SHA) that has taken over the work of the National Patient Safety Agency. The NHS SHA ensures that patient safety is at the heart of the NHS and builds on the learning and expertise developed by the NPSA, driving patient safety improvement.

Parliamentary and Health Service Ombudsman

www.ombudsman.org.uk/

The role of the Parliamentary and Health Service Ombudsman is to consider complaints that Government departments, a range of other public bodies in the UK and the NHS in England have not acted properly or fairly or have provided a poor service. The website provides access to the role of the Ombudsman and the legislation that supports it. You can also read about its vision and values and access the annual report.

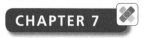
 # The University Setting

You may be new to the university setting and have never studied in the higher education sector before, or you may already have experienced how universities function when completing a course or degree at a higher education institution. As a student nurse in such an institution your course is very different to that being studied by the many other students. The NMC approves your programme of study and the institution you are in must be able to demonstrate that your programme meets standards set by the regulator as well as those set by other quality assurance agencies, such as the Quality Assurance Agency for Higher Education (QAA).

The QAA performs its duties to safeguard standards and improve the quality of UK higher education. The QAA conducts reviews of institutions and publishes reports that outline its findings. The reports produced by the QAA highlight good practice and contain recommendations to help improve quality. They also offer advice, guidance and support for UK universities, colleges and other institutions to provide the best possible student experience of higher education.

Chapter 1 of this book alerts you to the unique content of an undergraduate nursing programme: overall, the programme requires 50% theory (2300 hours) and 50% practice (2300 hours) (Nursing and Midwifery Council, 2010), undertaking person-centred activities such as the provision of hands-on care under supervision. These profession-specific requirements mean that your university experience will be very different to that of, say, an engineering student or a physiotherapy student.

The Student Nurse Toolkit: An Essential Guide for Surviving Your Course, First Edition. Ian Peate.
© 2013 John Wiley & Sons, Ltd. Published 2013 by John Wiley & Sons, Ltd.

To get the most out of your university experience and to make it an enjoyable and memorable one (for all the right reasons) you need to understand how the university system works. Some universities are centuries old and date back to as early as the twelfth century. Other universities are newer and indeed many came into being in the 1990s (see Table 7.1). Each university has its own idiosyncrasies, some dating back to medieval times.

Table 7.1 Categories of universities in the UK

Category	Comment
Ancient universities	For example Oxford, St Andrews, Cambridge and Glasgow
London, Durham and Wales	Chartered in the nineteenth century
Red-brick universities	Chartered before the twentieth century; large civic universities
Plate-glass universities	Universities chartered after 1966
The Open University	Established 1962, a distance learning university
New universities	Post-1992 universities, formed from polytechnics or colleges of higher education

In the UK universities have generally been instituted by Royal Charter, Act of Parliament or an instrument of government under the Education Reform Act 1988, in any case usually with Privy Council approval. Only these duly recognised bodies have the ability to award degrees of any kind. To be awarded the title 'university' an institution must meet certain criteria. These are assessed by the QAA acting on behalf of the Privy Council. The Privy Council has a responsibility, under the Further and Higher Education Act 1992, to approve the use of the word 'university' in the title of a higher education institution. Universities in the UK can be classified into six main categories, identified in Table 7.1.

Previously the majority of nurse education courses were provided in Schools of Nursing, usually attached to hospitals; for example, the Barnet School of Nursing was attached to and located within the grounds of the then Barnet General Hospital. The movement of Schools of Nursing (and as such nurse education) into institutions of higher education was not without its problems.

Each university has its own structure and way in which it is governed will differ to other universities; however, all will be subjected to in-depth quality assurance mechanisms (as mentioned, your nursing programme is subjected to quality assurance measures by the NMC and the QAA).

All universities in the UK undertake research and teaching, although the focus and balance of these activities varies. Some institutions concentrate primarily on teaching while others are more research-intensive. Universities also increasingly transfer knowledge out to businesses and other organisations, such as the NHS and the independent and voluntary sectors; this is known as knowledge transfer. Universities also seek to use their expertise and facilities to develop thriving social and business communities in their region; again, many of them are engaged with the local health and social care economy.

The university structure

It has to be noted that not all nursing programmes are offered by and in a university; the NMC use the term approved education institution (AEI). The Open University offers a number of programmes that lead to registration with the NMC upon successful completion of the programme through a modified distance learning route. University structures differ and you need to understand the structure that is applicable to the institution where you are studying if you are to get the most out of your programme.

The senior management team

The person who leads, manages or is in charge of the university is the Vice Chancellor. In some institutions this person may also be known as the Principal: she or he is the executive head of a university or college. In a company the equivalent would be the chief executive. Vice Chancellors provide strategic leadership and management; they also act as the key representative of the university externally. The role of the Vice Chancellor varies from university to university: in some the Vice Chancellor is largely a figurehead; in others they have more hands-on involvement. Roles and functions may include awarding degrees at graduation ceremonies and supporting fundraising efforts.

The governing body of the university is often known as the university council or board of governors and is responsible for the effective management and future development of the affairs of the institution. There may be a number Pro Vice Chancellors who assist the Vice Chancellor, each with their own specific portfolio; for example, research and enterprise, student affairs, quality assurance or international. Often universities are made up of faculties, which house schools or departments (see Figure 7.1). Faculties are usually headed by a Dean.

Vice Chancellor								
Pro Vice Chancellor Research and enterprise			Pro Vice Chancellor Student experience and international			Pro Vice Chancellor Quality assurance		
Dean of Faculty Business			Dean of Faculty Health			Dean of Faculty Law		
Head of School Accounting	Head of School Tourism	Head of School MBA	Head of School Nursing	Head of School Physiotherapy	Head of School Radiography	Head of School Maritime law	Head of School Medical law	Head of School Probation

Figure 7.1 The structure of a fictitious university.

The academic staff

Most of the academics teaching you will be either nurses or healthcare professionals allied to health, for example a doctor, physiotherapist or health advisor. The aim is to introduce you to a multidisciplinary approach. The majority of nurses who teach you will have a teaching qualification that is recordable with the NMC, meaning that they have undertaken an extra period of study to meet the criteria demanded by the NMC to have an annotation next to their name on the professional register. Most will have studied at undergraduate, postgraduate and doctoral level.

There are also other people who will teach you in the academic setting, such as consultant nurses, clinical nurse specialists and staff nurses. More and more expert patients (service users) are now involved in teaching too.

There is also a hierarchy in academia just as there is in the health and social care setting. Table 7.2 provides an overview of the typical hierarchy that may be seen in some schools of nursing (there are many different names for schools or departments that teach nursing as one aspect of their portfolio).

Table 7.2 A typical school structure (nursing)

Title	Role and function
Lecturer	A registered nurse. May have a recordable teaching qualification. Works on modules of study, link lecturer, has a group of personal tutees. Undertakes scholarly and research activity.
Senior Lecturer	A registered nurse. Has a recordable teaching qualification. Manages and works on modules of study, link lecturer, has a group of personal tutees. Takes on other school, faculty and university responsibilities. Undertakes scholarly and research activity.
Principal Lecturer/ Field Leader	A registered nurse. Has a recordable teaching qualification. Manages programmes of study, link lecturer, has a group of personal tutees. Manages a group of staff. Takes on other school, faculty and university responsibilities. Undertakes scholarly and research activity.
Associate/Deputy Head of School	A registered nurse. Has a recordable teaching qualification. Assists the Head of School. Links with senior external colleagues. May have a group of personal tutees. Manages a group of staff. Takes on other school, faculty and university responsibilities. Manages their own portfolio of activity, such as the student experience. Undertakes scholarly and research activity.

Table 7.2 *(continued)*

Title	Role and function
Head of School/Department	May be a registered nurse and if so will have a recordable teaching qualification. The Head of School is an Academic Manager. Assists the Dean of Faculty. Links with senior external colleagues. Is responsible for the overall quality of all programmes within the school as well as the student experience and income generation. Is overall responsible for performance of the school and has line-management responsibilities for staff. Takes on other senior school, faculty and university responsibilities. Undertakes scholarly and research activity. This job has an outward-facing aspect.

Professional administrative staff

No university or School of Nursing could survive without professional administrative staff. These are the people who make things happen. They support the academic staff and above all they support you, the student. The administrative staff are responsible (and this is not an exhaustive list) for:

- your application when it is submitted and how it is progressed,
- arranging and inviting you for interview for selection,
- dealing with your requests for accommodation,
- pointing you in the right direction with regards to issues such as finance and other aspects of support,
- keeping a record of your studies,
- organising examinations,
- organising the graduation ceremony,
- planning your learning experiences (placements),
- looking after you (your welfare).

Usually the professional administrative staff are managed by the Faculty Registrar.

Other support staff

Just as the university would come to a stand-still without the expert support provided by the professional administrative staff, so too would it and your studies flounder if it were not for other essential support services, such as:

- catering,
- estates,
- library and learning resource staff,
- technicians,
- careers support service,
- accommodation service,
- occupational health service,
- counselling service.

PEARLS OF WISDOM

It is important to know who is who and who does what, and to understand the basic structures in the university. If you have any concerns about any aspect of your programme of study you will then know who to turn to and at what level.

SECTION SUMMARY

University structures vary. Regardless of that structure, all universities have to conform to several standards to be able to award degrees. Understanding your university's structure will help you navigate the systems quickly and efficiently.

Student support services

Each university will have its own student services and they will all differ in the range of services they offer you. It is a good idea to learn what services are available to support you on your programme of study. You must also note that the university is not a school: it is concerned with the education of adults. Universities will not spoon-feed you, but they will support you, guide you and mentor you. You will not be spoon-fed as a staff nurse in charge of a busy 32-bed medical ward when you qualify. The onus is on you to seek help and support when you need it; hence the need to know what is available to you.

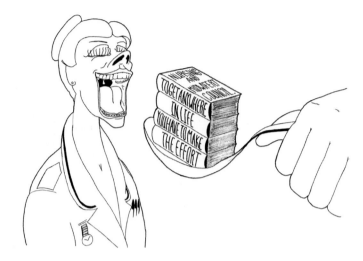

It is in a university's best interests to support you throughout your programme of study as it will wish to retain as many students as possible. Universities are keen to ensure that attrition rates (how many people drop out) is as low as possible, and so much effort is put into enhancing the student experience.

It has already been mentioned that support services such as the accommodation office and the occupational health service are there to help you. Use them if you need to, as they offer their services free of charge; they will not come looking for you, and you have to approach them if you need support. Seek support early on: it is unwise to let things fester, they will only become worse, you will worry and you will be unhappy.

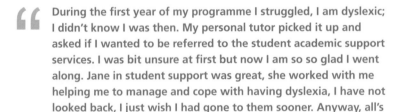

> During the first year of my programme I struggled, I am dyslexic; I didn't know I was then. My personal tutor picked it up and asked if I wanted to be referred to the student academic support services. I was bit unsure at first but now I am so so glad I went along. Jane in student support was great, she worked with me helping me to manage and cope with having dyslexia, I have not looked back, I just wish I had gone to them sooner. Anyway, all's well that ends well. *Jacob, third year student*

 ## The personal tutor

Each student, from the day they commence their programme (sometimes even before they start), should be allocated a personal tutor. Universities differ in the way they run the personal tutor system, but essentially the aim is to provide pastoral care. Some institutions also include academic support in this role.

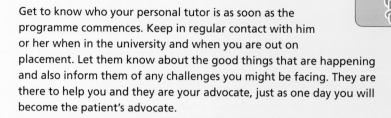

Get to know who your personal tutor is as soon as the programme commences. Keep in regular contact with him or her when in the university and when you are out on placement. Let them know about the good things that are happening and also inform them of any challenges you might be facing. They are there to help you and they are your advocate, just as one day you will become the patient's advocate.

Your personal tutor will usually have a background in the same field of nursing as your own; this person is a member of the programme team and will be involved in your academic progress.

> When I started the programme I was hesitant to go to 'teacher' but, I soon learned that he was the fount of all knowledge, had so much to offer me. My personal tutor willed me to succeed, he was inspirational. He has just sent off a reference for me for a job in the community – fingers crossed. *Mercy, finalist*

You will be encouraged to have regular contact with your personal tutor, who will offer you guidance and support, as well as monitoring your progress, ensuring that you are ready to progress between each stage of the programme. There are opportunities provided as the programme proceeds to enable you and your personal tutor, either on a one-to-one basis or in a small group, to meet regularly to enhance the integration of theory to practice.

> I meet with my personal tutor group individually and in small groups at least every semester. I encourage the students to come and see me, explaining to them that if they are having any problems it is best to share them and deal with them as soon as they arise. It is sad, however, that some students choose not to come to the sessions and it is usually those students who struggle. *Mary, personal tutor*

When you meet with your personal tutor this provides you with the opportunity to discuss your progress and seek feedback on the development of your personal development plan as the programme advances. Many universities insist that the personal development plan is a programme requirement; the onus is on the student to develop it with support from the personal tutor.

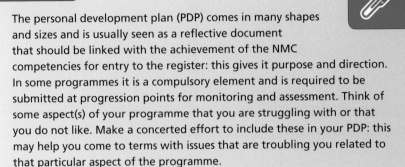

ACTIVITY 7.2

The personal development plan (PDP) comes in many shapes and sizes and is usually seen as a reflective document that should be linked with the achievement of the NMC competencies for entry to the register: this gives it purpose and direction. In some programmes it is a compulsory element and is required to be submitted at progression points for monitoring and assessment. Think of some aspect(s) of your programme that you are struggling with or that you do not like. Make a concerted effort to include these in your PDP: this may help you come to terms with issues that are troubling you related to that particular aspect of the programme.

Whenever you meet your personal tutor it is a good idea to keep a note/record of the interaction, what happened and what the outcome of the meeting was, and your personal tutor will also keep a record of the interaction. The personal tutor monitors your programme attendance (you also have a duty to monitor this) and normally compiles an end-of-programme reference in collaboration with you.

PEARLS OF WISDOM

Your personal tutor will most probably be a referee when you apply for your first staff nurse post. It is sensible, therefore, to keep them up to date with your progress throughout the programme, not just for the last month.

SECTION SUMMARY

There are a number of student support services at your disposal: use them, they have been put in place to support you, to make your life at university as enjoyable and as successful as possible. You have to use your initiative when considering these services: problems that you may experience are often best discussed with others and a solution worked out. The most influential person in the university may be your personal tutor, who will act as an advocate for you.

Student representative bodies

 ### The National Union of Students

The National Union of Students (NUS) is a national organisation that is the student voice. Membership of the NUS is voluntary; there are over 600 student unions in the UK and the NUS represents the interests of more than 7 million students. One of the many functions of the student union is to run student clubs and societies offering students help and advice. There is usually a fee payable to join the clubs or societies.

> I joined the university's debating society when I first started. I like a good debate and I have to say it has given me so much confidence at uni and when I'm on the wards I feel able to contribute more seriously. One of my module requirements is to take part in a debate and we get marked on it too. I did really well, all thanks to the students' union. I also met my boyfriend at a debate. *Siobhán, third year student*

 ### UNISON

UNISON is a trade union and has more than 25 000 student nurse members campaigning for a better deal for nursing students, and has run several campaigns around areas such as the bursary and accommodation.

As discussed, nursing students are in a unique position because they work on wards, in homes and in clinics but do not have employment rights; they are students yet do not adhere to a typical student calendar. Some nursing students work additional hours as healthcare assistants to manage the financial hardship they may face. This can be exhausting and potentially detrimental to their studies.

UNISON has much experience in representing students while they work as healthcare assistants throughout their training, providing assistance and advice.

 ### Royal College of Nursing

A professional body and trade union the Royal College of Nursing (RCN) supports students throughout their studies, representing their rights and offering advice. The RCN is the biggest professional union for nurses and nursing in the UK. The RCN describes its mission as one of representing nurses and nursing with the intention of promoting excellence in practice and shaping health policies.

The anatomy of a programme of study

A programme of study, for the purpose of this book, is the 3 years it takes you to complete your studies and then after successful completion apply for registration with the NMC. Sometimes programmes of study are also referred to as courses.

Regardless of the terminology used, there are certain requirements (standards) that all universities must be able to demonstrate that they have met to the NMC and QAA. Each programme must demonstrate that the student has studied the right number of academic credits at the right academic level before they can be given the academic award, the degree.

An undergraduate UK degree (a Bachelor of Science, BSc, or a Bachelor of Arts, BA) can be awarded with or without honours (Hons), with the class of an honours degree calculated on a weighted average mark of the student's assessed work. Each university has it own system but there will be similarities across institutions. Box 7.1 provides a list of the possible classifications with common abbreviations.

Box 7.1 Possible degree classifications

First class honours (1st)

Second class honours, upper division (2.i)

Second class honours, lower division (2.ii)

Third class honours (3rd)

Ordinary degree (Pass)

 ## The academic year

For nursing students the academic year is different to other students due to the statutory number of hours they are required to study (2300 hours). Summer vacation may also be shorter for the student nurse. The academic year is divided into terms or semesters (depending on your university). A semester can last for 16 weeks, and there are usually three semesters (two in some institutions) in the academic year. You will be provided with an academic calendar when you commence your studies and this will detail semester start and finish times, Christmas, Easter and summer holidays, as well as assessment dates.

Modular credits

In order to be awarded an undergraduate degree you must be able to demonstrate that you have achieved the right number of credits at the right academic level. A student studying full time for an honours degree must achieve 360 credits over the 3 years, 120 credits each year: these are broken down into levels (see Table 7.3).

Table 7.3 Academic credits

Year	Level	Number of credits
1	4 (sometimes called level 1)	120
2	5 (sometimes called level 2)	120
3	6 (sometimes called level 3)	120
Total		360

Each module (sometimes called a unit or a course) will be assigned a specific number of credits and the level will depend on the year in which you are studying that module. Modules combine to make a progamme. If, for example, all of your modules are worth 30 credits then during the 3 years of study you will need to complete 12 modules to get your degree. However, most institutions have a range of modular credit values (see Table 7.4).

Table 7.4 A typical overview of an undergraduate nursing honours degree with module credits and academic level

Year	Level	Subject	Credits (modular value)
1	4	Study skills	10
		Literature search	10
		Human development	20
		Health promotion	20
		Introduction to nursing	30
		Protecting vulnerable people	20
		Professional practice	10
Progression point 120			

Table 7.4 *(continued)*

Year	Level	Subject	Credits (modular value)
2	5	Professional practice	20
		Pathophysiology	20
		Medicines management	20
		Clinical decision making	30
		Managing care	10
		Public health	20
Progression point 120			
3	6	Nursing research	20
		Evaluating care	40
		Advanced decision making	20
		Leading care	10
		Advanced nursing skills	20
		Professional practice	10
Progression point 120			
Completion of programme: 360 academic credits			

You will note in Table 7.4 that there are progression points throughout the 3 years of study. There are important NMC criteria that have be evidenced and met at each progression point (end of years 1 and 2) of your programme (Nursing and Midwifery Council, 2010). The NMC has determined that you must complete all the requirements for the progression points of the programme.

Only in exceptional circumstances may you be permitted a further 12 weeks to meet all requirements if you have not proceeded at the progression point (i.e. not earned enough credits). Should you not be able to meet the criteria at the progression point you will be withdrawn from the programme or, at the discretion of the university, you may be put back a cohort to make good as stipulated by the NMC criteria.

 ## Teaching, learning and assessment

Your programme will be underpinned by an overall teaching, learning and assessment strategy, devised to enable you to grow into a skilled, knowledgeable, autonomous nursing practitioner who is able to deliver high-quality, evidence-based patient-centred care in a variety of health and social care settings. You will also be able to critically reflect on your actions and omissions (see Chapter 13) and engender the important concept of professional development and lifelong learning (see Chapter 18).

Your programme of study will have both theoretical and practical components associated with it and you will be assessed on both of these in the university and during your placements (learning opportunities). The range of assessments (also called the assessment diet) will vary according to the subject being assessed, the academic level and the number of credits for that module. Box 7.2 provides an overview of the various types of assessment strategy that may be used in your university.

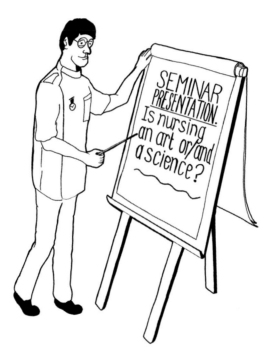

Many universities use two approaches to teaching and learning, employing blended learning along with an emphasis on learning in practice; the approaches are closely linked. During your programme you will be provided with a range of learning opportunities, which may include classroom learning, learning in the workplace, on-the-job learning and learning online at your pace. The advantage of online learning is that it can provide you with flexibility to undertake this learning

Box 7.2 Example of some assessment techniques that may form part of the assessment diet

All of the assessments below may be formatively or summatively assessed.

- Poster presentation
- Seminar presentation
- Short answer questions
- Multiple-choice questions
- Case study
- Literature review
- Essay
- Webinar/folio
- Personal development portfolio
- Clinical competencies
- Objective structured clinical examination

in an environment of your choice, on or off the university campus. A virtual learning environment, such as Blackboard, is often used to facilitate this. The integrated approach to learning and teaching is called blended learning and learning online is often referred to now as e-learning.

ACTIVITY 7.3

The ways in which we learn are varied. We all have preferred ways of learning with different learning styles. What is your learning style? There are a number of inventories available on the Internet that can help you identify your learning style. Cottrell (2008) has a number of useful exercises that will help you make the most out of the style you prefer, enabling you to broaden your study strengths.

Regardless of how you learn or how you are taught you must have the motivation to learn. You will have the support of your lecturers and mentors and you will be able to access a variety of learning materials and resources, including human resources. Importantly, learning is a shared responsibility between you, your lecturers, your mentors and those who are close to you. Lecturers can ensure that the right conditions are there to support your learning needs; you are expected to take responsibility for your learning, engaging fully in the process of learning.

The key issue with learning is that you are engaged with the process. Not all learning will take place in the classroom, or the workplace: you will be asked to access online materials so that you can undertake and participate in learning activities, access learning materials and contribute to online group discussions. Your university will help you access these materials, they will provide you with details such as the login procedure and your username and password as well as providing printed guides, websites, e-mail support and one-to-one contact. Box 7.3 provides a list of some examples of blended learning activities

Box 7.3 Examples of blended learning

- Lectures, presentations, guest speakers
- Simulation centre learning and role play
- Seminar and case study presentation
- Enquiry-based learning
- Assessing electronic resources
- One-to-one or group tutorials
- E-activities including online discussions using Skype
- Collaborative learning with other health and social care professions
- Reflective practice
- Support from peers and constructive feedback
- Self-directed study as an individual or in groups
- Action learning sets and supervision

Practice learning opportunities are discussed in Chapter 8.

Summary

The euphemism 'reading for a degree' is sometimes used when people mean, 'what are you studying?'. Studying for a degree has a great deal of reading associated with it and this is something you have to sign up to when you start the programme. You have a key role to play here: you will not be spoon-fed, you will be supported but the onus is on you, the adult learner.

Academic credits are awarded to you as you successfully complete various aspects of your programme. There are different modular values and the academic levels are associated with your year of study.

With a nursing degree 50% of your programme involves working with people. Teaching, learning and assessment strategies used in your university will have been devised to ensure that you are able to link theory to practice and practice to theory. Blended learning is an approach that is used widely and will form a part of every nursing degree.

To get the most out of your university experience you have to understand the university structure. Understanding academic and administrative processes will enable to you to direct any questions or challenges you are experiencing to the right person at the right level. There are many people who will be able to support you throughout the 3 years of your study; one central figure is your personal tutor.

 ## References

Cottrell, S. (2008) *The Study Skills Handbook*, 3rd edn. Palgrave, Basingstoke

Nursing and Midwifery Council (2010) *Pre Registration Nursing Education in the UK*. http://standards.nmc-uk.org/Documents/Pre-registration%20nursing%20education%20in%20UK%20FINAL%2006092010.pdf

 ## Resources

National Union of Students
www.nus.org.uk/
The NUS has a vision of being a pioneering, innovative and powerful campaigning organisation, the national voice of students. Its aim is to fight barriers to education and empower students to shape both a quality learning experience and the world around them, supporting influential, democratic and well-resourced student unions.

Quality Assurance Agency for Higher Education
www.qaa.ac.uk/Pages/default.aspx
The QAA is the UK authority on higher education standards and quality, aiming to safeguard standards and improve quality. It works to ensure that all students get the best possible educational experience.

Royal College of Nursing
www.rcn.org.uk/
See Resources section in Chapter 2

UNISON
www.unison.org.uk/
See Resources section in Chapter 2

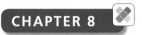

CHAPTER 8

Practice Learning Opportunities

- The practice setting
- Practice learning opportunities
- Teaching, learning and assessment
- Your role
- Getting the most of the practice placement

Fifty per cent of your programme takes place in the practice setting. The programme of study you have embarked on has been developed to make sure that you will be offered opportunities to meet the NMC standards for competency (Nursing and Midwifery Council, 2010) that are a requirement for you to register as a nurse in your chosen field. When undergraduate nursing programmes are planned, a range of people and organisations will be asked to take part in the development. Staff from the university will work closely with colleagues in nursing practice, patients and service users, and current nursing students (your peers) with the aim of ensuring that the programme is contemporary, responsive to the ever-changing needs of diverse health and social care services, is fit for purpose and is stimulating.

Clinical experience has always been an essential aspect of nursing education, preparing the student to be capable of 'doing' as well as 'knowing' the clinical principles in practice; in other words, becoming a knowledgeable doer. Clinical practice encourages students to use their critical thinking skills for problem solving.

It is in the practice arena where learning is applied and where your level of expertise is developed and honed with the aid of skilled practitioners, teachers, patients and their families. Learning and teaching are inextricably aligned with the development of your professional knowledge and competence.

The practice setting

The practice setting, sometimes called the clinical placement, the practice placement or the clinical experience, is crucial to the preparation of the student as they enter the workforce as a competent and autonomous practitioner and an

The Student Nurse Toolkit: An Essential Guide for Surviving Your Course, First Edition. Ian Peate.
© 2013 John Wiley & Sons, Ltd. Published 2013 by John Wiley & Sons, Ltd.

employee. Good-quality placements are required to ensure the ongoing development of the profession, without them students will not gain the required experience.

Nursing is a practice-based profession and, as would be expected, clinical education is an essential part of the undergraduate nursing curriculum. On the whole the quality of nurse education depends to a large extent on the quality of the clinical experience. It is essential that your clinical placements allow the application of theory to practice to occur.

Twentyman *et al.* (2006) comment on the importance of the clinical placement and how this can provide students with an opportunity to:

- observe role models,
- practice,
- develop skills associated with problem solving,
- reflect on what they see, hear and do.

There could have been many other things added to that list, for example:

- appreciate the realities of nursing,
- generate a feeling of belonging,
- working as part of a multidisciplinary team,
- develop all forms of communication skills,
- begin to understand the politics of nursing and healthcare,
- become more confident and competent with a range of clinical skills, environments and patients,
- appreciate that learning takes place in environments that are often unpredictable and unstructured, and that what occurs there can sometimes be overwhelming.

The environment of care is another phrase that is often used in association with or instead of the practice setting. The environment of care has wider inferences than the clinical area or the practice placement; it is a term used in the NMC code of conduct (Nursing and Midwifery Council, 2008a).

> I was working with a client with learning disabilities in a residential home and he needed to have an injection of iron. I had never given an injection before; we had practised in the simulation centre on the mannequins and oranges but I had never done it on a real live person. My mentor and I talked about me doing it with him supervising and supporting me. I was scared I might hurt the client; I might get it wrong, I might hit the sciatic nerve, we discussed all this. I did it and I did it well, I was chuffed, I used the experience to reflect on for the reflective aspect of my assessment.
> *Paul, first year learning disabilities student*

Recent changes in the delivery of healthcare show that a great deal of care now takes place outside of what used to be seen as traditional settings; for example, the hospital ward in the acute care trust. This shift for nursing, from the hospital to the community, focuses on prevention, acknowledging patients and the public as the drivers of their care. You must be aware of, and gain experience from, the changing needs of healthcare settings and the communities in which nurses (and you) work, responding to both current and future needs in contemporary health and social care settings.

The emphasis of a move to more community-based settings brings with it a shift in power (the power differential). It could be suggested that when a patient was admitted to a hospital ward the patient waited to be invited to the hospital (their admission letter) and while on the ward they were visitors. When the patient is being cared for in their own home, the nurse is the visitor. The nurse is being invited into the patient's home and the nurse must wait to be invited in, or may even be declined entry.

Carr (2008), a practice nurse who mentors students in general practice, notes that students are increasingly participating in health activities in diverse community settings and practice nurses and practice nursing can offer exceptional learning opportunities for students in any field of nursing. An understanding of community roles regardless of where the student is working can only enhance the quality and effectiveness of care; hence, a broad range of practice experiences are advocated.

The Royal College of Nursing (2006) suggests that an effective practice placement promotes learning and can help you to:

- meet the statutory and regulatory requirements,
- achieve the required learning outcomes and competencies according to the NMC requirements for entry on to the professional register,
- recognise the variety of learning opportunities available within health and social care environments,
- work in a wide range of rapidly and constantly changing health and social services,
- provide the full range of nursing care to patients,
- demonstrate and acknowledge the unpredictable and dynamic nature of the care setting as a learning environment within a multiprofessional approach to care,
- feel valued and safe in a culture that recognises and subscribes to the importance of adult learning,
- maintain your supernumerary status,
- work alongside mentors who are appropriately prepared, crafting a partnership with them,
- identify appropriate learning opportunities to meet your learning needs, generically and specifically,

🖐 use time effectively, providing opportunities to apply theory to practice and practice to theory,

🖐 reflect contemporary thinking in a dynamic and modern health and social care service to evaluate the efficacy of care provided, based on best available evidence,

🖐 continue to develop your competence in both interpersonal and practical skills,

🖐 provide truthful, evaluative feedback of your practice experiences,

🖐 develop and hone skills in information technology to access information within the placement area.

There is no dictum from the NMC related to the types of learning environment the student will experience, nor for how long they will be in the learning environment. This offers universities working with practitioners much scope to provide practice learning opportunities across a range of hospital, community and other settings. The NMC is keen for you to experience placements that reflect local and national trends associated with approaches to care delivery (Nursing and Midwifery Council, 2010).

SECTION SUMMARY

The quality of the clinical learning environment can have a positive or negative effect on the student experience. There are a number of factors that contribute to a positive learning experience and the student also has a role to play in making the learning experience a positive one. Practice education is an integral element of the undergraduate nursing curriculum. The practice experience should be one in which the student is permitted to apply the theory that underpins practice and vice versa.

 ## Practice learning opportunities

The various practice learning opportunities that will be made available to enable you to meet your programme outcomes will have been decided when the NMC and your university validated your programme of study. Universities and placement providers meet to discuss the range of practice learning opportunities available, and as such it is a joint responsibility.

Practice placements are where a nursing student applies their knowledge to practice, learns key skills and achieves the required competencies for registration (Royal College of Nursing, 2006). When learning in the contextual setting of clinical practice this will enable you to address many of the challenges and issues that are related to caring. Practice is where lifelong learning begins, and is promoted and enhanced.

ACTIVITY 8.1

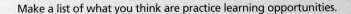

Make a list of what you think are practice learning opportunities.

How long was your list? It could, potentially, have been very long, as they could be anywhere where there are people. Some universities place the onus of finding practice learning opportunities on the student; most have a team of staff academics and professional administrators working with health and social care providers to supply a practice education circuit that will ensure that you receive the right experiences to ensure you develop confidence and competence in relation to the programme learning outcomes. Examples of practice learning opportunities are outlined in Table 8.1.

Table 8.1 Examples of practice learning opportunities

Field	Examples of potential practice opportunities
Child	Child health community team (community child health nurse)
	Acute care settings (hospitals, accident and emergency)
	School nursing
	Health visiting
	Voluntary and independent sectors
	Hospice
Learning disability	Residential and community care settings
	Adult education settings
	Social care settings
	Occupational health department
	School nursing
	Health visiting
	Voluntary and independent sectors
	Independent living homes
	Supported living and family homes
	Treatment and assessment services
	Challenging behaviour units
Mental health	Acute mental health services (including accident and emergency)
	Community psychiatric services (community psychiatric nurse)
	Practice nursing
	Occupational health department
	Prisons and places of detention
	Probation service
	Health visiting
	Voluntary and independent sectors
	Treatment and assessment services

Table 8.1 *(continued)*

Field	Examples of potential practice opportunities
Adult	Community team (community nursing) Acute care settings (hospitals) Ambulatory day care Nursing and residential homes School nursing Health visiting Practice nursing Occupational health department Voluntary and independent sectors Military settings Prisons and places of detention

You may have noted from the list in Table 8.1 that there are many overlaps; for example, you may be working in a prison setting as a student of adult nursing and you may also be working with students from the mental health field. Likewise, as a learning disability student you may have been allocated to work with a school nurse and on that placement there may also be a student from the field of child nursing at the same school. This provides an example of how generic and specialist aspects of the nurse's role will cross over and impact on each other.

PEARLS OF WISDOM

You should have an open mind when you are working in the various practice placements: think outside of the box and apply what you are learning, seeing and doing in a broad manner. For example, if you are working with a health visitor apply the principles of public health to all care settings.

Other additional practice learning opportunities may include:

- ☥ formal teaching by university staff and staff in the practice area or simulation centre,
- ☥ ward rounds with teachers/link lecturers,
- ☥ attending a case conference or practice meeting,
- ☥ supervision sessions with the personal tutor/link tutor.

It is also important to note that in the practice setting you will be working with students from other health and social care professions, such as physiotherapy, social work, speech and language therapy, pre-hospital emergency care, medicine and midwifery. When this occurs you should seize the opportunity and share experiences and use these experiences when you are reflecting on practice (see Chapter 13).

 I was working on a brain injury unit, my first placement, and it was fab. There were students from my university who were doing occupational therapy, physiotherapy and speech. We all got together as part of our interprofessional learning module and we did a great multidisciplinary case study presentation when we got back to university. It made me think and understand how it really is all about team working. *Rashiela, first year student*

SECTION SUMMARY

Nursing practice occurs wherever there are people. What used to be considered as the 'traditional' education circuit no longer exists. Students now experience how nursing is practised in a number of diverse services that reflect how care is delivered in contemporary health and social care settings. There are learning practice opportunities available in each field of nursing with a degree of helpful overlap.

Teaching, learning and assessment

This heading appears in Chapter 7, and there is refers to the university setting. This aspect of the chapter focuses on teaching, learning and assessing in the practice setting. It is important to note that you cannot split the two, the theory and the practice, because you are required to integrate the theoretical components of the programme to the realities of nursing.

Practice learning is also known by a number of other names; for example, on-the-job learning, work-based learning and the apprenticeship working model (observing experienced colleagues at work). Regardless of the words used the aim is to expose you, safely, to how nurses work and interact with the people they care for so that over time you will become confident and competent. It is also essential that the people you are caring for are also safe and as such you are required to practice under supervision at all times. As you progress into your second and third years less direct supervision is required. This allows you to demonstrate that you can work more independently, with less direct supervision, in a safe and increasingly confident manner, extending your knowledge and skills (Nursing and Midwifery Council, 2010).

Teaching and learning

From the outset it has been acknowledged that the clinical experience is often one of the most anxiety-producing aspects of the nursing programme. The things that can cause you undue anxiety can include:

- the placement being your first placement (initial clinical anxiety),
- lack of clinical exposure,
- unfamiliar areas,
- unwelcoming staff,
- challenging patients,
- fear of making mistakes,
- worrying about giving the wrong information to patients,
- fear of being assessed and failing.

Being aware of these issues may make you feel more settled in so far as you should understand that the anxiety you may feel may also be experienced by your peers. You are not alone.

PEARLS OF WISDOM

The golden rule is, if you are unhappy on your practice placement, you must make this known as soon as you can. Speak to your mentor, link lecturer or personal tutor. If you are unhappy this could be reflected in the care you deliver or the relationships you have with others.

Conversely, if you are having a great time let people know that as well.

A range of people may teach you when working in the practice setting, these include:

- your peers (other nursing and healthcare students),
- your mentor (your teacher),
- other nursing staff (consultant nurses, clinical nurse specialists),
- other healthcare professionals (dieticians, podiatrists, midwives, doctors),
- the patient and their families,
- representatives for medical devices and pharmaceutical companies.

When learning in the workplace (wherever that may be) the workplace becomes the learning environment and is filled with many opportunities from which you can learn. The workplace can be seen as an 'opportunistic setting' for teaching, but many of the opportunities are unpredictable, random and spontaneous and will be very much patient-dependent, with a lot of the teaching and learning relying on chance. Regardless of how the learning opportunities arise, you should see them all as possible learning events and take from them as much as you can. Circumstantial factors have the potential to impact significantly on the learning opportunities available and the teaching provided; sometimes this can place additional stress on both you and the teacher.

> ### PEARLS OF WISDOM
>
> Try not to be a shy wallflower. Make known your learning needs and seize the opportunity to learn; put yourself forward when opportunities arise. For example, if there is a chance to escort a patient to theatre then ask to take part.

You and the teacher may have to juggle with a number of competing demands; for example, from the patient and their family, the organisation in which you work, professional requirements (such as those demanded by the NMC) and other healthcare professionals. Remember that your teacher (mentor/facilitator) works with a number of students, coming from a number of backgrounds, and each one of them will have their own unique learning style (see Chapter 7); they too have to provide safe and effective nursing care to patients.

Sharples (2011) makes the important observation that despite being surrounded by potential learning opportunities, learning will not take place automatically, as if by osmosis. You have to take some of the responsibility for learning.

Nurses tend to be practical or experiential learners (Kolb, 1984); they usually learn best from doing something as opposed to reading about it. So it is likely that the following approaches will be used:

- the theory you learn will be easy to understand and assimilated if it is related to everyday life,
- clinical practice or real-life scenarios will bring facts and theory alive,
- group work will be used to pool ideas and allow you to learn from each other,
- you will be encouraged to explore 'what if' situations or case studies where a problem can be solved using the information you have been learning,
- visual media such as video, pictures and diagrams will be used to describe theory and concepts as well as encouraging recall.

Bearing the above in mind you need to ensure that you plan (as far as you can) what it is you are going to learn. This should begin prior to being allocated to the practice placement.

Assessment

Assessment is a broad term that is used for a set of processes that measure the outcomes of your learning in relation to knowledge acquired, the understanding developed and the skills gained. Assessors make judgements against a set of criteria about your performance and a variety of methods are used to used to do this, for example, observation, questioning and testimonies (Hand, 2006).

A variety of names are used when referring to the people who will assess and support you in practice, such as teacher, mentor, assessor, preceptor and practice educator. The English National Board for Nursing, Midwifery and Health Visiting (ENB and DH, 2001) made a decision in an attempt to ensure consistency that the term mentor was to be used.

When a formal assessment takes place this assesses your learning at regular points against defined criteria. The assessment will provide you with information that will help you identify where your learning has been effective and where you might need to improve. Teachers can also use assessment results as one of the means to measure learners' progress and identify and agree learning needs.

Each university has its own ways of assessing clinical competence: some use practice assessment documents and others use a skills handbook. A portfolio of evidence, regardless of the type of document used, must comply with the NMC standards (Nursing and Midwifery Council, 2008b, 2010). Your university will help you understand the assessment document and what is required of you at different stages of the programme. It also ensures that the people assessing you understand the programme and the curriculum, and it does this through updates and workshops.

The competence of all nurses has to be assessed with the explicit aim of protecting the public, ensuring quality of education and maintaining credibility of the profession. Assessing your competence is more than performing a given task or ticking a checklist: the public have to be assured that the assessment is valid and reliable and that processes are in place to demonstrate fairness, transparency and robustness. Standards have been established by the Nursing and Midwifery Council (2008b), assessments that take place ensure that those standards are met. It is the quality of this assessment that protects the overall reputation of professionals.

PEARLS OF WISDOM

You will be required on your practice placement to take part in a preliminary, mid and final interview where your progress will be discussed with you. These important milestones are time-specific and you have to ensure that they occur when they should during the placement. If there is a danger that the timing is slipping make this known to your mentor first and then your link lecturer.

SECTION SUMMARY

Teaching, learning and assessing in clinical practice must conform to standards laid down by the NMC as well as your university. The processes used must be valid and reliable, fair, transparent and robust. There are a number of opportunities that are available to you to develop your cognitive and psychomotor skills. You must practice under supervision with the aim of ensuring that the people you care for are safe.

Getting the most out of clinical learning opportunities: roles and responsibilities

It may seem rather daunting, given all of the things going on in the learning environment, how you can do it all. As well as recognising your own responsibilities you must also recognise those of your higher education institution and the various placement providers. By understanding these you will know where and who to turn to should you need any support or guidance. There are many stakeholders who have a role to play in ensuring the experience you have is a positive one. The key stakeholders include:

- you (the student),
- patients/clients cared for in all sectors where healthcare is provided,
- the NHS, independent and voluntary sectors,
- your university and staff such as personal tutors, programme directors, cohort leaders and subject/module/academic leaders/link lecturers,
- service providers, those who are part of the tripartite arrangements, your university and the commissioning body. These include the clinical team, mentors, lecturer practitioners and practice educators/facilitators.

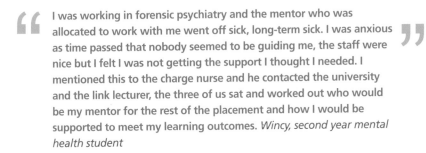

I was working in forensic psychiatry and the mentor who was allocated to work with me went off sick, long-term sick. I was anxious as time passed that nobody seemed to be guiding me, the staff were nice but I felt I was not getting the support I thought I needed. I mentioned this to the charge nurse and he contacted the university and the link lecturer, the three of us sat and worked out who would be my mentor for the rest of the placement and how I would be supported to meet my learning outcomes. *Wincy, second year mental health student*

Planning is your best friend and a close second is maintaining your energy levels and motivation. Planning should begin prior to being allocated to the practice placement. Box 8.1 provides you with some suggestions to which you should give serious consideration, prior to, during and after your placement.

Box 8.1 Your responsibilities before, during and after a practice placement

Prior to the placement you must ensure the following.

- Develop an understanding of the student handbook that explains your programme of study as well as the Student Charter issued by your university. You will have been given these when you commenced your programme. These handbooks will identify the joint obligations between you and the university, highlighting the university's responsibility to meet the requirements of the programme (a kind of contract).
- Read and refer to the student handbooks that are related to your specific programme of study. There will be information in the handbooks that will relate to your practice placements, including the teaching and assessment of practice.
- Understand the purpose of the practice placement experience, ensuring you are clear about the expectations of the service provider in that you are there to learn.
- Check that you understand the specific expectations of the placement; you can ask the placement office or link lecturer prior to attending.
- Make contact with the placement.
- Behave professionally with regard to time keeping, attitude and image, and ensure you abide to uniform policy.
- Respect and maintain confidentiality.
- Strive to engage in effective communication with patients, clients, personal tutors, mentors and link personnel from the placement and the university.
- Understand how it is you are going to meet your learning needs, using learning tools, assessment, learning contracts, learning logs and reflective diaries.
- Identify what your specific learning needs are, working towards the achievement of knowledge and the required outcomes and competencies.

During placement you have a responsibility to do the following.

- Be forthcoming in seeking out experiences for your level of practice and competence, enlisting the support of your mentor.
- Show willingness to work as part of the team when delivering safe patient care.
- Devise ways of expressing your needs, adopting a questioning, reflective approach to learning as a member of the multidisciplinary team.
- Make use of your mentor for direction and support, enabling you to achieve your learning outcomes and completing your practice assessments.
- Request help from appropriate clinical managers or link lecturer if your relationship with your mentor is failing to enable you to achieve the learning outcomes.
- Work to ensure that clinical skills required at the various stages in the programme are attempted while under the supervision of a skilled practitioner, with comments provided by you both.
- Make use of the learning opportunities outside the practice placements and, when the opportunity arises, work with specialist practitioners.
- Recognise the role of professionals within other contexts of the organisation or community.
- Offer and receive constructive feedback.
- Reflect on your development with the intention of increasing self-awareness, confidence and competence.

When the placement is over you have the following responsibilities.
- Assess and evaluate your achievements, considering what you enjoyed and benefited from during the practice placement.
- Provide an evaluation of the placement itself.
- Prepare for meetings with your personal tutor and for discussion in the classroom.
- Continue with regular contact with your personal tutor, keeping them informed of any worries or problems you might have.
- Submit and forward to the university, in a timely manner, all practice placement documentation and assessments of practice.

Source: data from Royal College of Nursing (2006).

Box 8.1 outlines your responsibilities for making the practice placement a success. In Box 8.2 the responsibilities of your university are detailed.

Box 8.2 The university's responsibilities to ensure a positive practice experience

- Monitor both the capacity and quality of all practice placements to meet statutory and professional body requirements.
- Ensure that practice placements meet all standards for the programme validated by the university.
- Carry out a joint annual audit of all practice placements.
- Make responses and take action following audit concerning the capacity and quality of the practice learning environment.
- Ensure there are sufficient numbers of link lecturers and lecturer practitioners available to support students and staff in placements.
- Provide students access to support structures while in their practice placement, with details of contact numbers in student handbooks.
- Keep a live register of mentors, ensuring there is the availability for the numbers of students allocated to the placement at any one time.
- Strive to ensure that the placement opportunities identified are conducive to the student's level of experience to facilitate and build their confidence in practice.
- Keep mentors informed when changes are made in the curriculum, programmes or modules.
- Ensure placement areas have documentation reflecting student requirements at every stage of the programme of study.
- Facilitate effective communication networks between the university and the practice placement.
- Provide an effective system of jointly monitoring feedback about students' practice placement experiences.
- Provide a system of informing students when actions have been implemented to improve practice placements, where concern was noted.

Source: data from Royal College of Nursing (2006).

Personal tutors, mentors and service provides should work in such a way that they too assume responsibility for providing a learning environment that is appropriate and meaningful, meeting the needs of students and enabling them to achieve programme learning outcomes.

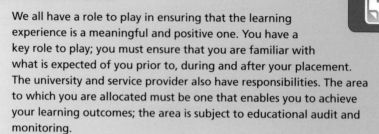

SECTION SUMMARY

We all have a role to play in ensuring that the learning experience is a meaningful and positive one. You have a key role to play; you must ensure that you are familiar with what is expected of you prior to, during and after your placement. The university and service provider also have responsibilities. The area to which you are allocated must be one that enables you to achieve your learning outcomes; the area is subject to educational audit and monitoring.

 Supernumerary practice

As a student you will be supernumerary when you attend your practice placements. There are many ways of interpreting what supernumerary means and this often causes much angst for students, practitioners and academics. The Nursing and Midwifery Council (2010) have determined that supernumerary means that as a student you will not, as part of your programme, be contracted by any person or body to provide nursing care. The rationale underpinning this is to ensure (as far as is possible) that students are free to learn as opposed to being counted as a part of the nursing establishment. What it does not mean is that students are free to disengage in the provision of care or that they only 'observe' practice.

> I was due to commence my first night duty, I was so anxious, I know it sounds stupid but I thought, 'what happens if I fall asleep?' Well, there was no chance of that; it was as busy on nights as it was on days, but in different ways.
> *Lenny, first year student*

SECTION SUMMARY

Supernumerary status was introduced to enable you to be free to learn; it is not about abdicating your responsibilities as a student of nursing.

Simulation centre

Most universities have state-of-the-art simulation centres offering you experiences that are as near to real life as possible. You will spend time in the simulation centre with the intention of ensuring that you acquire knowledge and practice skills in a safe and controlled environment prior to experiencing the real world of health and social care. The work you do in the simulation centre will dovetail with the work you do in the classroom. Some simulation centres allow you to access their resources in addition to timetabled activity, providing you with opportunities to brush up on skills you may be unsure of or need to revise.

 Summary

An integral aspect of becoming a nurse is being able to perform with competence in the practice setting. Learning in practice is as important as learning at the university. There are a variety of placement opportunities available; the important thing about these diverse placements is that they will facilitate you achieving your learning outcomes. You and the people who provide the learning opportunities (the university and service providers) all have a responsibility, a tripartite responsibility, to ensure that the placement is a meaningful and enjoyable experience.

You will be assessed during the placement where mentors will assess your knowledge, skills and attitude against set criteria and standards issued by the NMC and the university. Assessment is continuous and should be fair, transparent and robust. There will be a number of people available to offer you support during your placement but you must take a significant amount of responsibility for your own learning. Feedback is provided to you on a regular basis with the intention of helping you develop personally and professionally.

 References

Carr, J. (2008) Mentoring student nurses in the practice. *Practice Nursing* 19(9), 465–7

ENB and DH (2001) *Preparation of Mentors and Teachers – A New Framework of Guidance.* English National Board for Nursing, Midwifery and Health Visiting and Department of Health, London

Hand, H. (2006) Assessment of learning in clinical practice. *Nursing Standard* 21(4), 48–56

Kolb, D. (1984) *Experiential Learning: Experience as the Source of Learning and Development.* Prentice Hall, New Jersey

Nursing and Midwifery Council (2008a) *The Code: Standards of Conduct, Performance and Ethics for Nurses and Midwives.* Nursing and Midwifery Council, London

Nursing and Midwifery Council (2008b) *Standards to Support Learning and Assessment in Practice.* Nursing and Midwifery Council, London

Nursing and Midwifery Council (2010) *Pre Registration Nursing Education in the UK.* http://standards.nmc-uk.org/Documents/Pre-registration%20nursing%20education%20in%20UK%20FINAL%2006092010.pdf

Royal College of Nursing (2006) *Helping Students get the Best From Their Practice Placement.* RCN, London

Sharples, K. (2011) *Successful Practice Learning for Nursing Students.* Learning Matters, Exeter

Twentyman, M., Eaton, E. and Henderson, A. (2006) Enhancing support for nursing students in the clinical setting. *Nursing Times* 102(14), 35

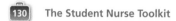 **Resources**

Higher Education Academy

www.heacademy.ac.uk/

The HEA has a subject centre that is concerned with health sciences and practice. There are a number of useful links; for example, a link to a special interest group, the practice learning and support group.

NHS Careers

www.nhscareers.nhs.uk/

Provides insight into a variety of NHS careers available, as well as offering information on the work that different nurses and other healthcare professionals undertake.

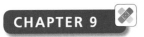

CHAPTER 9

The Nursing Elective

WHAT THIS CHAPTER CONTAINS

- The purpose of the elective
- Preparing for the elective
- Finding funding
- How to arrange an elective
- Getting the most out of the elective

The elective is not a new concept. Elective studies have been part of nursing and medical curricula for a number of years. The way an elective placement is managed and undertaken differs with each university. Much of the discussion in Chapters 7 and 8 will be applicable to this chapter and the nursing elective. Your motivation and your efforts will have a big impact on a successful and enjoyable outcome.

The world is your oyster when it comes to nursing electives and you have almost unlimited opportunities to experience something that is truly unique. Some students will travel overseas and experience the delivery of nursing care in another country, whereas some will use the opportunity to work in an area of nursing in which they one day hope to gain employment after completing their studies.

The purpose of the nursing elective

Nursing electives can provide the student nurse with a range of new opportunities to experience and observe care from different perspectives in the UK or abroad. For you to get the most out of the elective placement, wherever that may be, you have to plan it with much precision, in advance: it must be planned like a military manoeuvre. You need to spend time and give thought to preparing for this activity. There are a number of resources (human and material) that are available to help you with the planning. Beginning to plan early for the event can make it much more successful, whereas rushing or leaving it to the last minute and taking chances is not to be recommended.

The Student Nurse Toolkit: An Essential Guide for Surviving Your Course, First Edition. Ian Peate.
© 2013 John Wiley & Sons, Ltd. Published 2013 by John Wiley & Sons, Ltd.

The duration of an elective is at the discretion of the university: it can be a 3–8-week period of work experience and is usually spent in another country but can also be in a UK health or social care setting. Many students (but not all) choose to travel overseas, with developing countries being popular destinations. Worldwide teaching hospitals, non-governmental organisations (NGO), charities and religious organisations are often receptive to student electives. Some of these organisations may charge a fee to cover expenses and to help support other projects (the amount varies). Generally, the elective experience is made available to students in their final year of study.

There are several important things you need to consider. For example, the funding of the elective event needs to be thought about early on in the planning stages (the earlier the better) if it is likely to be a problem. Funding includes more than just the cost of a flight. You will have to consider the practical issues, such as insurance cover, the need for an honorary contract, the safety of the region you are thinking of visiting, the need for immunisations, and travel and other documents. The elective opportunity has the potential to provide you with a unique experience, and in some instances a once-in-a-lifetime experience, a chance to delve deeper into a specific area of interest as well as potentially experiencing the provision of health and social care through an alternative lens.

Depending on your university an elective can be an optional module in itself, not a compulsory part of your programme of study. The elective can be thought of as a short sub-programme of the broader nursing curriculum, with the student taking the lead in determining the subject and method of study. From a philosophical perspective the elective is based on the premise that you usually know what it is you want to learn and that you are best placed to discriminate from what is on offer in light of your ultimate career objectives. The intention is to promote creativity and innovation so that within a loose set of guidelines you set your own aims and objectives as well as determine the ways you are to achieve them. Your personal tutor/programme leader acts as a facilitator rather than the source of all knowledge. Electives, therefore, are clearly about learning but they are not all about teaching. Using electives often means that the teacher has to get out of the driving seat, taking on the role of passenger, and hand the steering wheel to the student.

> " Being given the opportunity to undertake an elective can be quite daunting: you are the one leading the initiative, you have to be really organised, devise aims and objectives, take calculated risks and make serious decisions. The planning experience really spurred me on though; it motivated me to look at something in depth that I was really interested in. *Kaylee, third year student*

The work required to organise and succeed in the elective prepares the student for real-world working, reacting to the demands of fluid, ever-changing and dynamic environments, and encouraging the student to become an autonomous thinker. Electives are normally in a subject area that is not available as part of a nursing curriculum but are be subject (nursing)-related and will give you an excellent opportunity to broaden your studies. Some programmes do not allow students to take electives because of the way the curriculum has been organised; you should check with your personal tutor or the programme leader in your school or department.

The way the elective is organised will be dependent on programme requirements: if your school does permit you to take an elective this means you can or must choose experiences outside of the learning opportunities that are available in your programme of study (practice or theory). If the elective is classed as a module of study further consideration needs to be given to the number of modular credits you can or must study. Again, you should seek advice and support from your programme leader (or their equivalent). If an elective opportunity is available to you then this will be stated in your programme handbook or on the university's website.

One of the purposes of a nursing elective is to provide insight into areas of nursing not elaborated upon in the regular curriculum or to provide an in-depth investigation of a specific content area. There may be restrictions to prevent you taking an elective that is too closely related to what is available on your programme. For example, you may want to delve deeper into the practicalities of electroconvulsive therapy. However, if there is an opportunity to do this using current placement opportunities on your current practice placement circuit then it may not be allowed as an elective. There would be no point in encouraging you to seek this experience elsewhere when it is available to you locally.

ACTIVITY 9.1

Make a list of potential nursing electives. When you have completed the list look at the pros and cons of each item on your list. This might help you focus and think of ideas in a more realistic way.

Elective idea	Pros	Cons

One aim of the nursing elective is to provide you with a vision of the broader scope of nursing. You need to consider where it has been and where it may be going. The success of the elective largely depends upon the amount of effort and time that you are prepared to put into it.

Clark-Callister and Harmer-Cox (2006) noted that when international clinical nursing electives are undertaken they can have an impact on the personal and professional lives of nurses. Box 9.1 highlights the benefits of experiencing an international experience.

Box 9.1 Some of the benefits associated with undertaking an international nursing elective

> ᷉ Increasing understanding of other cultures and peoples
> ᷉ Increasing understanding of global sociopolitical and health issues
> ᷉ Increasing commitment to making a difference
> ᷉ Experiencing personal and professional growth
> ᷉ Contributing to professional development in the host country
> ᷉ Making interpersonal connections
> ᷉ Developing cultural competence

Source: Clark-Callister and Harmer-Cox (2006).

Clark-Callister and Harmer-Cox (2006) refer to the nursing elective from an international perspective, but just as much learning can take place if you choose to undertake your elective in the UK, nationally or locally.

> **For my elective I was really lucky to be working with a health visitor in Cheshire who worked with a group of travellers; my objective was to gain insight in how families interact and manage their health. I was totally amazed how different we all are as people. We all have our own cultures even within cultures. I learned more about me and my family than I did about the travellers and their families.**
> *Joanna, third year child student*

It is wrong to think of the health of the UK in isolation from the rest of the world: UK health is concerned with global health. There are several benefits when UK healthcare providers become involved in helping to improve global health. The Department of Health (2007a, 2007b) suggests that by becoming involved in global health partnerships the UK will be able to learn more about how to meet its own health needs. There is an opportunity to broaden the education of UK healthcare professionals and the possibility of developing and enhancing relationships across the globe, with us all working as one to address global health threats.

SECTION SUMMARY

Understanding the rationale for nursing electives can help you plan more effectively. Each university will have its own systems and processes in place to which you must adhere. Nursing electives can take place in the UK (locally or nationally) as well as abroad. You are strongly advised to seek advice from the most appropriate people as early as possible concerning your ideas for a nursing elective.

Preparing for the nursing elective

Other chapters in this book have encouraged you to get to know who is who in the university; the same has to be said for the elective placement. In some organisations electives are managed by one person – the elective tutor – whereas in other universities the elective experience may be coordinated through your personal tutor or the programme tutor. Whoever it is, you need to know who to contact and the correct processes that are to be used. You should attend any sessions the university organise about the elective. These may be briefing sessions, and their objective is for you to learn about the processes and to begin to crystallise your ideas and start to make plans.

During the preparatory phase share your ideas, discuss issues that concern you and be realistic in setting your aims and objectives. Your personal tutor or the person responsible for coordinating elective experiences will be asking you a number of probing questions that will determine how well thought through your ideas are. By engaging in frank and open discussions both of you will be able to come up with ways of finding alternatives or devising original approaches to any apparent hiccoughs.

PEARLS OF WISDOM

You should bear in mind that while your elective coordinator will encourage you and your ideas, she or he is not naïve. They will be alert to any ulterior motives you may have; for example, a desire to delve deeper into occupational health services in a hotel in Mexico may be viewed with suspicion. The primary objective must be convincing, genuine and honestly fulfilled.

When you have thought through carefully and realistically about the elective you wish to pursue there will no doubt be some form of paperwork to complete. The paperwork will be specific to your university but in general it will require you to demonstrate how you will meet your learning outcomes, provide evidence of attendance and complete reflective accounts of your experiences (this may be classified as part of your coursework and you may be marked on it). You must ensure that all of the administrative procedures are complete.

Other practical aspects will include things like whether you need to wear a uniform, what type of uniform it will be and who will pay for it. You should consider contacting UNISON or a professional organisation such as the Royal College of Nursing, the international offices of which may be able to put you in touch with, or provide you with details of, national nursing associations in other countries.

Returning to the nursing process (see Chapter 5), consider the four phases (approach 1 in Table 5.1). You can apply these to the way you approach preparing for your elective placement (see Table 9.1).

Table 9.1 The elective experience using a nursing process approach

Phase	Action
Assess	Gather all the information you need, carry out a literature search and engage in personal communications with others.
Plan	Plan well in advance, anticipate the opportunities and challenges that you may face, set realistic and achievable goals. Formulate aims and objectives.
Implement	Do it, enjoy it, learn from it and tell people about it: disseminate your findings.
Evaluate	If required, undertake a reflective account of your activities, carry out an evaluation of the experience, which will help others who are also undertaking an elective.

SECTION SUMMARY

For a nursing elective to be a success it is essential that you make preparations well in advance. You must know to whom to turn to plan your elective placement. Use a systematic approach to planning your elective to ensure that all bases have been covered.

 Finding and funding an elective

Some universities will pay all of your funding for an elective, but generally you will be required to self-fund your elective and as such it is advantageous to start planning well in advance. International electives will be considerably more costly than national or locally based ones, but remember that home electives can also incur costs. The funding aspect of the elective should be one of the first things you consider.

Begin by planning an initial budget, and do this as early as possible, even before you know what the exact costs will be. This can be adapted and changed as you progress with the planning but it will give you a solid foundation from which to work. It also has a number of advantages:

- it demonstrates to potential sponsors that you are organised,
- it will give you an idea of what type of elective is financially realistic for you.

The main items you will need to budget for can be found in Box 9.2.

Box 9.2 Key items to budget for on an international elective

- Travel, including flights and in-country travel
- Visas: you should go the UK Foreign Office website, which provides comprehensive travel advice by country as well as links for all international embassies in the UK. Visas need to be paid for and costs vary depending on the type of visa and the duration.
- Travel insurance is vital; it covers not only your belongings but also emergency medical treatment and repatriation if needed.
- Professional indemnity insurance: you may need this and you must find out if this is the case. Professional indemnity insurance is additional to travel insurance.
- Accommodation costs vary. It could be a home-stay with a local family, a room at the university or hospital where the elective is taking place, bed and breakfast, a hotel or a hostel.
- Fees: some organisations may charge for the elective. Find out in advance and, if a fee is payable, ask how much it will be.
- Day-to-day living costs; for example, food and water (sustenance)
- Medical supplies, a medical pack for your own needs: this may include needles and syringes and if so you might need a covering note for Customs and Excise explaining why you are taking these items with you.
- Pre-travel immunisations will need to be paid for as most GP practices charge for them.
- Malaria prophylaxis costs will vary depending on type of tablets you take.
- Personal spending money will depend on how much holiday travel you are planning as well as what part of the world you will be in (it will be cheaper in parts of Asia and Africa than Australia or America).

 Funding opportunities

There are funding opportunities available but you have to search them out. Funding can come from private, public and individual sources that are willing to support student electives.

PEARLS OF WISDOM

When it comes to funding, be creative and daring. The maxim 'if you don't ask, you don't get' is very true.

When you begin your search for funding opportunities you may find that some organisations make certain stipulations with regards to who may or may not be considered for funding. In some instances you may only be considered for funding if, for example, you live within a certain locale (catchment area) or if you are from a specific community group (for example, the Jewish community). Others may only offer assistance if you are from a black or minority ethnic background.

The financial assistance that is available may cover all of your expenses or it may only cover certain aspects, such as travel, subsistence or accommodation costs. Regardless of the amount you might receive every penny will help ease the expense of an elective. If you receive funds in advance it is a good idea to make sure that you keep them separate from the rest of your money; you should consider putting them in a separate bank account. Box 9.2 can form the basis of your financial plan but be realistic: if you underestimate costs it could detract from the experience of the elective.

ACTIVITY 9.2

Return to Box 9.2 and see if there are any other budgeting considerations you need to add to this list. Did you think of the price of a 10-year passport and how long it may take to get one?

There are a number of publications available that help those who are seeking to raise money from grant-making trusts and foundations (see, for example, French *et al.* 2010). These publications provide clear descriptions of trusts' grant-making policies and practices, including contact details and advice to applicants.

SECTION SUMMARY

Issues surrounding the funding aspects of the elective should be one of the first things you consider. There are some public, private and individual sources available that may fund all or some aspects of your elective. You should pay particular attention to the criteria laid down by sponsors as some of them have certain stipulations.

Making contact

Planning should begin early, as some locations are very popular and they can only host a finite number of students. Have plan B in place and if your first choice is not available start putting plan B into action immediately: do not be disheartened.

Make initial contact with your chosen placement in a professional and positive way, stating why they should take you, the benefits you will get from the elective and the possible gains to their organisation and the advantages this will make to the profession and the impact it could have on patient care. Follow up the informal contact with a formal approach detailing clearly what was agreed, clarifying what you want to gain from the placement prior to, during and after it has occurred.

Risk assessment

Discuss your thoughts with your personal tutor or the elective placement coordinator and ensure that all processes have been adhered to. You may be required to undertake a risk assessment associated with the place you are visiting (this can also apply to some venues in the UK as well as overseas). The risk assessment may require you to address the following issues:

- appropriate local health and safety induction,
- the need for safety equipment,
- research into country culture,
- suitable clothing for modesty,
- details of the accommodation you will be staying at,
- immunisation requirements,
- personal indemnity and travel insurance,
- correct visas, and letter of invitation from host organisation,
- details from the Foreign Office safety advice for the country you are visiting,
- name and contact details of an emergency contact while you are outside UK.

Imagine you are going on holiday to Nepal and that you want to scale Mount Everest. Undertake a risk assessment for this once-in-a-lifetime holiday. The risk assessment should focus on your own health and safety.

SECTION SUMMARY

You should make contact as soon as you can with the people who will be hosting your elective placement and have plan B in place in case your first choice is not available.
A risk assessment may be required prior to undertaking the elective; this may apply equally to the UK and overseas.

 ## Getting the most out of your elective placement

To get the most out of your elective, this section provides you with a few pointers, irrespective of whether your placement is in the UK or abroad.

Have in place an honorary contract and keep copies; sometimes this is known as a memorandum of agreement. The contract will provide details concerning whether or not you are allowed to work hands on under supervision or if they will only permit you to be an observer without a formal contract of employment.

> From the day we had our first briefing on preparing for the elective, half way into the second year, I kept a folder with all of my elective information in it, adding to it as different things were needed, such as my MRSA screen. Being this organised meant that I was really quick off the mark when contacting the place I wanted to go to. I got the placement I wanted at a hospice in Cornwall. I have just got a job at that hospice. *Nicola, third year student*

Some hosts will require you to provide a written occupational health clearance document detailing your immunisation status. Some countries require you to provide a chest X-ray; you may need to be inoculated against diseases such as hepatitis A and B. It is not unusual for you to be required to provide evidence of your HIV and hepatitis C status. There may be a requirement to undergo a meti-cillin-resistant *Staphylococcus aureus* (MRSA) screen; you must be able to provide the evidence of the screening. All of this must be done in a timely manner. The

Department of Health has published a helpful booklet concerning health advice for travellers (Department of Health, 2006).

While working away you must ensure that due consideration is given to your own personal health and safety. Take antimalarial tablets if they have been advised by the practice nurse; you might also need to pack a mosquito net to sleep under as well as applying insect repellent. A high-factor sun block can help to prevent heat stroke and sunburn, as can common-sense actions such as drinking extra fluids to prevent dehydration and wearing protective clothing such as a hat and sunglasses. The use of protective clothing will also apply should you be travelling to colder climates. Be streetwise while travelling (just as you would be at home). This means do not flaunt electronic technology such as an Android or iPad tablet, mobile telephones, excessive jewellery or large amounts of cash.

There are some host organisations that will require criminal record screening. They may be prepared to accept the Criminal Record Bureau screening that your university has carried out on you: you need to find out about this.

Table 9.2 provides a checklist, and you can add to and delete items from this list to match your needs.

Table 9.2 A checklist for your elective

Item	✓
University administrative paper work complete:	
application form	
accommodation form	
learning contract	
honorary contract	
Contact details of elective placement coordinator	
Criminal Record Bureau statement	
Practice assessment documentation with personal learning outcomes	
Practice timesheets	
Occupational health clearance documentation	
Protective clothing (uniform)	
Health supplies (antimalarials, condoms, sunblock)	
Tickets, transport details	
Insurances	
Risk-assessment form	
Contact details of key people	
Travel guide	

Summary

Central to the philosophy of the nursing elective is the belief that nursing students have individual specific needs, bringing with them a wealth of experience and knowledge. Students often know what it is they want to learn and how to go about this. The nursing curriculum is enriched by the inclusion of nursing electives as this enhances innovation and creativity for all participants. Undertaking a nursing elective has the potential to encourage a strong sense of self-confidence along with the cultivation of autonomous thinking. Those who participate in nursing electives may have more to contribute to the understanding and the creation of culturally sensitive care environments as a result of being exposed to other ways of living, thinking and working. Making an effort to understand health and social care from a global perspective can help health and social care globally, nationally and locally.

Risk assessments and adherence to occupational health requirements will be required prior to starting out on the elective. Getting the most out of your elective means that you need to know who is who at your university and, specifically, who is responsible for coordinating the elective event. Use a checklist to ensure that all requirements have been adhered to.

For the elective experience to be a success planning and forethought are prerequisites, and don't forget to enjoy yourself.

References

Clark-Callister, L. and Harmer-Cox, A. (2006) International clinical nursing electives. *Nursing and Health Sciences* 8(2), 95–102

Department of Health (2006) *Health Advice for Travellers*. HMSO, London

Department of Health (2007a) *Health is Global: Proposals for a UK Contribution to Health in Developing Countries. Summary and Recommendations*. HMSO, London

Department of Health (2007b) *Global Health Partnerships: The UK Contribution to Health in Developing Countries*. www.dh.gov.uk/en/Publicationsandstatistics/Publications/PublicationsPolicyAndGuidance/DH_065374

French, A., Craver, J. and Smyth, J. (2010) *The Guide to the Major Trusts 2010/11*, vol 2. Directory of Social Change, Liverpool

Resources

Foreign and Commonwealth Office

www.fco.gov.uk/en/travel-and-living-abroad/travel-advice-by-country/

This website provides an A to Z of country advice, full of useful information for countries throughout the world. It also provides information concerning safety for the country you will be visiting.

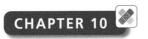

CHAPTER 10

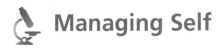 **Managing Self**

WHAT THIS CHAPTER CONTAINS

- Personal values and beliefs
- Self-awareness and assessment
- Managing self and interpersonal skills

Managing yourself encapsulates a number of important components. You need to look inwards, develop the important skills associated with self-awareness and you may need to challenge yourself about things that you do not like. You might even have to change some of your behaviours so that you are able work more effectively with people and in teams.

Turton (2012) considers that self-management can be the starting point of leadership and management. These activities form part of the NMC's standards for pre-registration nurse education (Nursing and Midwifery Council, 2010) and reflect your personal and professional development. The moment you begin your programme of study you will be embarking on a lifelong journey that will hone the skills that are associated with self-management and as such leadership and management.

There are many skills that you need to work on to address and perfect self-management; for example, you will need to consider your appearance, your attitude and the way you demonstrate respect and compassion. As nurses we need to be viewed as competent, knowledgeable and compassionate in the care we provide and professional in the way we behave. There may be times when we would really like to say how we feel, but we know that doing so would be unkind and disrespectful. In a sense, this means that we need to always 'act' the part of a nurse and one way of doing this is to develop our 'inside' and 'outside' voices. It is through this type of self-management that you become a great nurse, mastering the inside and outside voices.

The Student Nurse Toolkit: An Essential Guide for Surviving Your Course, First Edition. Ian Peate.
© 2013 John Wiley & Sons, Ltd. Published 2013 by John Wiley & Sons, Ltd.

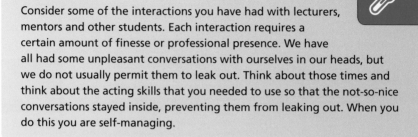

Consider some of the interactions you have had with lecturers, mentors and other students. Each interaction requires a certain amount of finesse or professional presence. We have all had some unpleasant conversations with ourselves in our heads, but we do not usually permit them to leak out. Think about those times and think about the acting skills that you needed to use so that the not-so-nice conversations stayed inside, preventing them from leaking out. When you do this you are self-managing.

Turton (2012) notes that self-management skills range from the fundamental requirements of reliability and attitude to more professional issues of effective communication, risk management and the performance of complex clinical skills. The start of the journey to managing self has to be to examine your value and belief systems. We all have them, but we need to acknowledge them and know what they are and how they can impact on others.

Values and beliefs

Each one of us is a unique being and we all have our own personal values and beliefs that have been shaped by a number of factors. Carvalho *et al.* (2012) state that each person's morals and ethics develop over a lifetime and originate from a variety of things that are valued. Values are central to the way in which we define ourselves as individuals and so too is our sense of who we are.

Think about your values and beliefs, and write them down as a list. Then list what you think shaped the values and beliefs that you hold.

In your list, did you include things such as your culture, family, education, religion, the law and your personal experiences? All of these can impact on what we value and what we believe in.

Values are related to our personal principles, morals and ideals; that is, what we consider to be important. It is not easy to define what exactly values are. Beliefs are related to the things in which an individual has faith, such as their religious beliefs. Beliefs may not necessarily be based on fact. The most important thing to remember is that not everyone subscribes to the same values and beliefs: people have different moral perspectives and aspire to different ideas, not everyone is of the same religion or even subscribes to a religion. Understanding and accepting this can help you begin to provide care that is patient-centred, respectful and effective. When you consider your own value and belief system carefully, and you are clear about the concepts that you value, you will begin to understand why a particular lecturer, mentor, peer or patient affects you in a certain way (Carvalho *et al.*, 2012). All of these things are associated with ethics: morality and ethics deal with how humans treat other beings.

Your values and beliefs have the power to influence your behaviour. It is wise to remember that the NMC's code of professional conduct (Nursing and Midwifery Council, 2008) makes clear that nurses must respect the people they care for and act in a non-judgemental way. Nurses should be ready to share mutual beliefs, values and emotions without any criticism or judgement.

PEARLS OF WISDOM

Of course we all make judgements, all of the time, it is what we do with the judgements as opposed to having them that matters: it is how you behave professionally that is important.

The value base associated with nursing has been articulated by the Royal College of Nursing (2003), which suggests that nursing is founded on ethical values which respect the dignity, autonomy and individuality of human beings, the privileged nurse–patient relationship and the acknowledgment of personal accountability for decisions and actions that nurses take. The values expressed here are the cornerstone of the NMC *Code* (Nursing and Midwifery Council 2008) as well as other written codes of ethics, supported by a process of professional regulation.

When caring for people, a number of issues may arise that may challenge your own personally held values and beliefs and you may well be required to make decisions that oppose you own beliefs. You have to counteract this by remembering that all nurses must provide care that is anti-discriminatory in nature and with the patient's best interests at heart.

Along with values and beliefs go assumptions and attitudes. Attitudes are based upon our beliefs and values arising from our experiences. They are judgements about how to act and they exert a strong influence over our physical and emotional behaviour. Bear in mind that attitudes emerge from the experiences we have, meaning that there is potential to change them as a result of new experiences.

Whenever you are being assessed, particularly in relation to nursing care, the examiner will be judging you based on number of things but, most importantly, will focus on three areas:

1 your knowledge (what you know),
2 your skills (how you perform an activity),
3 your attitude (how you behave).

SECTION SUMMARY

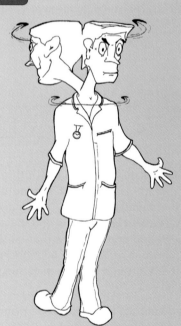

Your values and beliefs are aspects of personal growth and it is important for you to understand what yours are. All of us have an internalised system of values and beliefs that has grown throughout our lives. We use these values and beliefs to both guide our actions and behaviour and help us to form our attitudes towards different things. Self-aware people are consciously (or unconsciously) aware of their own values, the things that are important to them and the essence of what they believe in. As nurses the care we provide must be patient-centred and non-judgemental.

Self-awareness

Self-awareness has long been seen as essential for the professional nurse with the view that it will lead to greater competence. Being self-aware can help you self-manage and when you are self-managing effectively you will be more able to provide safe, efficient patient-centred care. Being aware of your own actions or of the effect these have on others is associated with being self-aware. It is essential in many aspects of the work you do as a nurse. Self-reflection is the tool that is most useful for developing self-awareness (there is more about reflective practice in Chapter 13).

Crowell (2011) suggests one skill that nurses have to develop is the ability to meta-communicate with yourself, meaning to be able to think about how you are think-ing and observe how you are acting in a given situation. Being in touch with your mind, bodily sensations and emotions are central to being self-aware.

One of the many challenges nurses will face is how to integrate their own val-ues and beliefs appropriately into their everyday professional practice. The thera-peutic nurse–patient relationship provides many opportunities to engage mutual feelings, recognise strengths, address fears, make choices known, instill faith and strive to achieve goals. Yet at the same time the nurse should be aware and sensi-tive to any conflicts, personal dramas and experiences of the patient.

The nurse can offer much support, including spiritual and moral support, which is a valuable way to promote well-being and contribute to helping the patient to cope better with any difficult life events. To do this effectively the nurse must be self-aware as well as attempting to understand the needs of the patient. An holis-tic approach acknowledges the person's health and illness from all perspectives, including the nurse's own.

Nurses are in a privileged position, and can impact on and influence patient behav-iour. Care provided on a daily basis and the relationship that has been created on mutual trust make it possible for the development of a special connection, the therapeutic relationship that provides an opportunity for both parties to exchange their insights and views. It is essential that the nurse understands what such an approach entails; equally important is to acknowledge that the relationship, despite its closeness, also has boundaries.

Self-awareness is a dynamic, transformative process of self. Self-awareness is the use of self-insights and presence knowingly to guide behaviour that is honest and genuine with the intention of creating a healing interpersonal environment (Eckroth-Bucher, 2010).

PEARLS OF WISDOM

The three Rs
- Respect yourself
- Respect others
- Responsibility for your actions

The Johari window

Using the Johari window can help us develop the issue of self-awareness further. You may have already been introduced to the Johari window during your programme of study. The Johari window was developed in the 1950s by two psychologists, Joseph Luft and Harry Ingham (Luft and Ingham, 1955); hence Joe Harry, or Johari. According to Luft (1970) the self arises out of self-appraisal and the appraisal of others, representing each individual's unique pattern of values, attitudes, beliefs, emotions, behaviours and needs. Self-awareness is the recognition of these aspects and understanding about their impact on the self and others. The Johari window provides a representation of the self and is a tool that can be used to increase self-awareness.

The tool also has a place in helping you to reflect on your interpersonal relationships at work and in social situations. However, like all tools and models they can only help or assist you: they do not give you the answer to all of your problems or challenges.

> We did the Johari window when we first arrived at the university, it was so uncomfortable, at least for a while, and now I am at the end of the second year it's much easier. We use the Johari window every 6 months to reflect and compare. The findings are sometimes not what you want to hear but at least you know where you are, and then you work to put things right.
> *Maribelle, second year student*

There are four squares (quadrants) in the Johari window. Each of the squares represents the knowledge, skills, values, attitudes and feelings of an individual (these components have already been discussed in this chapter). The areas depicted by the square reflect to what extent this information is shared or hidden from others or from yourself.

The four Johari squares:

1 what is known by you about you and is also known by others: the open area, open self, free area, free self or 'the arena',
2 what is unknown by you about you but which others know: blind area, blind self or 'blind spot',
3 what you know about yourself that others do not know: hidden area, hidden self, avoided area, avoided self or 'facade',
4 what is unknown by you about you and is also unknown by others: unknown area or unknown self.

Figure 10.1 provides a visual description of the Johari window.

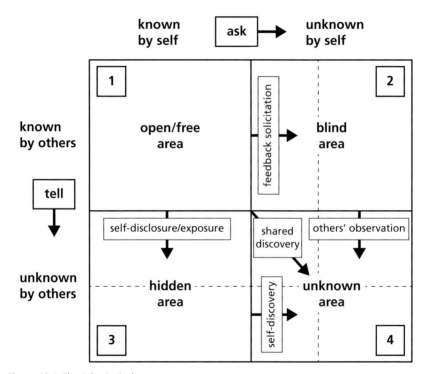

Figure 10.1 The Johari window.

Using the tool

Open area When using the Johari tool the aim is to work on developing or expanding the 'open' square. Opening up this area will help nurses improve their learning and professional development. As nurses we should be striving to communicate better with patients, work effectively as a team member and seek respect from the people we work with. Expanding this square, opening it up further, offers a greater space for effective communication, real, authentic behaviour and better-quality relationships within the numerous group dynamics experienced daily.

Blind area The intention is to grow and develop into the blind area; this can be achieved through seeking honest feedback from other members in the group and other people you work with. The type of feedback received can range from formal performance meetings (when you are on a placement) with a mentor or link lecturer to informal chats with your friends or others in your student group. You may have been working in a particular care area for some time and you may have a larger blind area because you have not received valuable (or valid) feedback, or it could be that despite feedback that was given to you, you have not taken it on board. As you develop in confidence and competence there is a danger that this blind area gets pushed back: your knowledge base increases, your knowledge of policies and procedures develops and you may not visit the blind area as often as you could. By asking a lot of questions and seeking out commentary on your performance you will be able to delve deeper into this square, improving your self-awareness.

Hidden area Expansion into the hidden area requires careful attention. When looking at this square you are required to undertake much disclosure and this necessitates an environment of trust. It requires you to be brave and to expose some of your inner self, and sometimes this is not easy. You are entitled to have your own secrets, thoughts and feelings that you keep to yourself; this is expected. It might be inappropriate, and the consequences could be disastrous, if we all revealed our deepest thoughts and feelings in full to everyone else on every occasion. Appropriate disclosure of information can improve our shared understanding and our effectiveness within a group. This can be a case of admitting to what we do not know as opposed to what we do. As a novice nurse or an advanced beginner you may have a larger hidden area than a more experienced nurse; in practice a first year student nurse is sure to have a larger hidden area than a third year. As that nurse becomes more comfortable and feels safer within the environment then their knowledge, skills and attitudes will begin to be disclosed to others in the group and at this stage new learning begins and the journey from novice to advanced beginner to competent nurse begins (Benner, 1984). All of us, novice nurses and expert nurses, may have large unknown areas, and this can be due to a number of reasons. For example, our current level of knowledge or lack of exposure to experiences means that we have not (yet) been exposed to the learning that will enable us to know more about the environment in which we work.

> " At the start of the course, my tutor said to us, 'it is always OK not to know something. It is never OK to pretend that you do if you don't.' *Franz, first year student*

Unknown area As we delve deeper, pushing back the boundaries of our blind and hidden areas, we can reveal elements of our interpersonal relationships that none of us were aware of, and they can emerge and become self-evident. The boundaries here expand as a result of a combination of self-discovery and a willingness and openness to seek and accept help from others, such as your peers, mentors, patients and lecturers. This help is often called feedback.

You may be asked to give feedback. Be careful in the way you give feedback. You can cause incredible offence if you offer personal feedback to someone who is not used to it. Be sensitive and start gradually.

ACTIVITY 10.3

Self-awareness provides you with a skill in establishing relationships with people who may have different values, beliefs, attitudes and principles than you. You achieve this through the therapeutic use of self. What does your own window look like? In this activity you are encouraged to think of what kinds of activities you might use to open up your own space. The aim is to open the window and let in some fresh air.

Use the window below, adjusting the sizes to reflect how open, blind, hidden or unknown you are feeling now compared to when you started your nursing programme. Use the windows to make a comparison: reflect on who you are now compared to who you were 5 years ago. You can do this alone; you may wish to share it with your personal tutor when you have a tutorial. Doing this can help you when you are required to ask patients about who they are, which might give you some insight into how they feel when somebody is curious about their lives.

Look at the different sizes of the squares and think about how open, blind, hidden or unknown you feel to yourself.

1. Open	2. Blind
3. Hidden	4. Unknown

When you have done the activity think about the following.

1 Reflect on how you were prior to your nursing programme (remember you were asked to compare): have you become more open?

2 Look at square 2 and consider whether there is anything that other people see about you that you do not notice or that you find hard to see yourself.

3 Be brave: what is hidden about you? What don't you know (yet)?

4 What else needs to be discovered about you? You might need to do some guessing here.

5 How did it feel delving deeper? Was it easier to do the exercise alone or with another person?

SECTION SUMMARY

Self-awareness can help the nurse to understand his or her own emotions, motivations and behaviours and as such have a better understanding of how these factors may impact on the nurse–patient relationship. Self-awareness, in its simplest form, can be defined as knowing one's self: it is about recognising your strengths and limitations, and acknowledging, accepting and confronting/challenging who we are and what we feel. The Johari window is one tool that can help you delve deeper and explore further; however, it is no more than a tool for you to reflect on.

Being self-aware provides you with the opportunity to begin to understand your own emotions, motivations and behaviours and therefore develop a better understanding of how these factors can impact on the nurse/patient relationship.

I am now a senior sister on a cardiac intensive care unit. To this day I remember how stupid I felt as a student. Now I tell all the students that come to our unit, no matter how stupid you feel, all the nurses in this hospital were once in your shoes. Be patient with yourself: as you learn more your confidence will grow, be kind to yourself and you will be kind to your patients.

Soma, senior sister in cardiac intensive care

 ## Managing self and personal skills

A common theme throughout this text has been that effective communication underpins all we do as student nurses and registered nurses. The discussions in this chapter reiterate this. Becoming self-aware is the first step towards personal development. The use of the Johari window is one way of identifying who you are and then putting plans in place to change (if change is needed). Sometimes interpersonal skills are also referred to as social skills, people skills, soft skills or life skills: these terms can often be broader and can also refer to other skills.

You already possess interpersonal skills. You have some idea of how others are likely to react to what you say, how you say it and what you do, and also how these actions make others and yourself feel. When you spend more effort and give more time to working, thinking and practising them then you can enhance them to their full potential. It is worthwhile spending time developing these skills as good interpersonal skills can improve many facets of your life, both personally and professionally.

Interpersonal skills are the life skills that we use every day to communicate and interact with other people, individually as well as in groups. They not only include how we communicate with others, but also our confidence and our ability to listen and understand. Problem solving, decision making and personal stress management are also considered interpersonal skills so, as you can see, they are wider than just 'communication'.

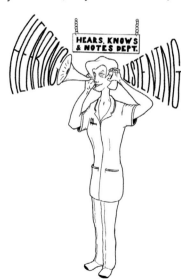

Those people who have and are able to demonstrate that they have strong interpersonal skills are generally more successful in their professional and personal lives. They are perceived as being calmer, more confident and charismatic; other people often find these qualities engaging or appealing. Here are some important interpersonal skills that you can work on and improve:

- listening,
- communication (including verbal and nonverbal communication),
- assertiveness,
- decision making,
- problem solving,
- stress management.

Listening skills

It is important to know that just because you hear someone you are not necessarily listening: listening is not the same as hearing. Hearing refers to the sounds that are heard, but listening entails more than that, it involves focus. When you are listening you are paying attention to more than the story: how it is being told, the use of the language being used and the voice as well as how the other person uses their body. Listening is about being aware of the verbal and nonverbal messages. Your ability to listen effectively will be dependent upon on the degree to which you have perceived and understood these messages. Box 10.1 provides you with some tips that may help you become a more effective listener.

Box 10.1 Some tips for developing your listening skills

Stop talking and prepare yourself to listen
Focus on the speaker. Put other things out of your mind. Remember you are listening and the other person is speaking. After the other person has finished speaking you may need to seek clarification.

Put the speaker at ease and remove distractions
Help the speaker to feel free to speak. Consider their needs and concerns. Use gestures such as nodding or utterances to encourage them to continue. Focus on what the person is saying to you, on what is being said; do not shuffle papers, look out of the window or doodle. Avoid unnecessary interruptions.

Empathise and be patient
Make every effort to understand the other person's point of view and consider issues from the other person's perspective. Have no preconceived ideas. If the speaker pauses (even a long pause), this does not automatically mean that they have finished. Never finish a sentence for someone.

Avoid any personal prejudice
Make every effort to be impartial. Do not become irritated and do not let the other person's habits or mannerisms distract you from what they may be really saying.

Listen to the tone
The volume and tone both add to what somebody is saying.

Wait and watch for nonverbal communication
Observe the person's gestures, facial expressions and eye movements. All of these can all be important.

Communication (including verbal and nonverbal communication)

The key elements essential in communication are discussed in Chapter 6. Box 10.2 provides a recap on some of the essential points.

Box 10.2 Some key essentials associated with communication

The communicators
There must be at least two people involved for any communication to occur. Communication is more than a one-way process where one person sends the message and the other receives it. Communication is nearly always a complex, two-way process, involving people who are sending and receiving messages to and from each other. Communication is an interactive process.

The message
The message is composed of more than the speech used or the information being sent, it is also about the nonverbal messages that are being exchanged; for example:
- facial expressions,
- tone of voice,
- gestures,
- body language.

Nonverbal behaviour has the ability to transmit additional information about the spoken message. It can expose more about emotional attitudes that may underlie the content of speech.

Noise
Noise refers to anything that changes the message, so that what is being received is different from what is meant by the speaker. It has a special meaning in communication theory. Although physical noise – for example, background sounds – can interfere with communication, there are other factors that are considered to be 'noise', such as the use of:
- jargon,
- inappropriate body language,
- inattention,
- disinterest,
- cultural differences.

Box 10.2 *(continued)*

Feedback

Messages the receiver returns can be considered feedback, allowing the sender to know how accurately the message has been received, also the receiver's reaction. The receiver can also respond to the unintentional and the intentional message. Kinds of feedback vary from direct verbal statements, such as 'Repeat that again, I did not understand', to subtle facial expressions or changes in posture indicating to the sender that the receiver feels uncomfortable with the message. Feedback permits the sender to regulate, adapt or repeat the message with the intention of improving communication.

Context

All communication is context-dependent; that it, is influenced by the context in which it occurs. The situational context of where the interaction occurs – for example, in a GP's surgery or in the patient's own home – must be considered. So too must the roles, responsibilities and relative status of the participants, such as the student nurse and the mentor.

Channel

The physical means by which a message is transferred from one person to another is the channel. In face-to-face conversation the channels used are speech and vision, yet when using the telephone the channel is limited to speech alone.

 ## Assertiveness

Being assertive means that you are able to express your feelings, wishes, needs and desires appropriately, which is an important interpersonal skill. Assertiveness can help you to express yourself in a clear, open and rational way, without jeopardising your own rights or those of others when interacting personally or professionally.

Acting in an assertive way can enable you to act in your own best interests, to stand up for yourself without unwarranted anxiety, to express true feelings in a comfortable way and to express your personal rights without denying the rights of others.

 ## Decision making

Decision making has been highlighted in the NMC's standards for pre-registration nursing (Nursing and Midwifery Council 2010); making decisions can be complex. Nurses have to make complex decisions on a daily basis, despite all best intentions and regardless of the effort that is put into making a decision. Some decisions made will be the wrong ones.

When nurses make decisions they choose between two or more possible courses of action. It should be remembered that there may not always be a correct decision arising from the available choices. There may have been a better choice that was not considered or the right information may not have been available at the time.

When arriving at an effective decision this can be made using either intuition or reasoning (Benner, 1984), and often a combination of both approaches is used. Regardless of the method used, it is helpful to use a systematic approach whenever possible. Approaches vary from simple rules of thumb to extremely complex procedures that are underpinned by a sound evidence base.

 ## Problem solving

There are two features in common in problem solving:

1 goals: the desire to achieve some objective, avoiding a particular situation or event;
2 barriers: if there were no barriers associated with achieving a goal, there would be no problem. Problem solving includes overcoming the barriers or obstacles that hinder the immediate achievement of goals.

Effective problem solving usually involves a number of steps (consider the nursing process in Chapter 5 and how that was used as a problem-solving approach):

- problem recognition: identifying and acknowledging that there is a problem, identifying the kind of the problem, defining the problem;
- structuring: a period of fact-finding, observing, inspecting and developing a clear picture of the problem;
- seeking potential solutions: producing a variety of possible courses of action; at this stage there will be little attempt to evaluate them;
- making a decision: careful analysis of the different possible courses of action and then selecting the best solution for implementation;
- implementation: accepting and carrying out the chosen course of action (the doing stage);
- evaluating/monitoring/seeking feedback: reviewing the outcomes of problem solving over a period of time, seeking feedback as to the success of the outcomes of the chosen solution, the decision made.

 ## Stress management

There are number of sources of stress. Many people suffer from symptoms of stress at some time in their lives. Sources of stress can include:

- personal stress that may be caused by the nature of your work, or significant life events such as getting married, getting divorced or the death of a spouse or partner;
- family stress or stressed friends, which may in turn affect you;
- workplace stress – that is, stress in your colleagues – which may also affect you.

The effects of stress can be unpleasant at the very least, and they can also make a person physically and psychologically unwell. People find different events and situations less or more stressful. A range of events or situations are acutely stressful to most people, and many would agree that major life events, for example, losing a job or having money problems, would be stressful for anyone. Many of the most stressful situations are unplanned changes in personal circumstances. Take measures to know what stresses affect you, and the means by which they can be avoided, confronted, managed and reduced.

Stress can be caused by events and there are certain situations that can lead to an individual feeling stressed, although the amount of stress will depend, among other things, on that person's ability to cope, their coping strategies. Our environment can also cause us stress; for example, noise, crowded wards, ward layout, poor lighting, air pollution or other external factors are things that we may have no control over and which can cause us to feel anxious and irritable. Stress is now commonplace in personal and professional lives. Box 10.3 provides some pointers for coping with stress.

Box 10.3 Tips for coping with stress

Talk to someone
Just talking to someone about how you feel may help. You can choose who you talk to: your personal tutor, a friend, the counselling service, your practice nurse. Talking works by taking your mind off your stressful thoughts or by releasing pent-up tension. Stress has the ability to cloud your judgement and prevent you from seeing things clearly. Talking things through can help you find solutions to your stress and put problems into perspective.

Engage in physical activity
Hormones such as adrenaline and cortisol are increased when you experience stressful situations. Physical exercise can be used to metabolise the excessive stress hormones, restoring your body and mind to a calmer, more relaxed state. If you are feeling stressed and tense, a brisk walk in the fresh air may help. Incorporate some physical activity into your daily routine on a regular basis, before or after work. Regular physical activity can also improve the quality of your sleep.

Relaxation techniques
There are many tried and tested relaxation techniques that can help to reduce stress: try a few and see what works best for you. You may find it difficult to relax at first, but don't worry: relaxation is a skill that needs to be learned and improves with practice.

Sleep
Try to get more sleep; lack of sleep is a significant cause of stress. Stress can also interrupt sleep as thoughts keep spinning through your head, preventing you from relaxing enough to fall asleep. Maximise your relaxation prior to going to sleep. Make sure that your bedroom is a calm haven, free of those things that cause you stress. Avoid caffeine during the evening and also excessive alcohol as they can lead

to disturbed sleep. Try to stop doing any mentally demanding work several hours before going to bed; this gives your brain time to calm down. Aim to go to bed at about the same time each day so that your mind and body get used to the routine.

Keep a stress diary

Keeping a stress diary for a few weeks is an effective stress-management tool; it can help you become more aware of situations that cause you to become stressed.

Record the date, time and place of each stressful episode, noting what you were doing, who you were with and how you felt, physically and emotionally. Rate each stressful episode (on a 1–10 scale) and use the diary to understand what the triggers are that cause you stress and how effective you are in stressful situations. This has the potential to enable you to avoid such situations and develop better coping mechanisms.

Take control

Learning how to find solutions to your problems will help you feel more in control and consequently lower your stress levels. Write down the problem causing you concern and devise as many possible solutions as you can. Note the good and bad points of each one and choose the best solution. Write down each step that needs to be taken as part of the solution; for example:

- what will be done,
- how will it be done,
- when will it be done,
- who is involved,
- where will it take place.

Time management

Managing your time is a skill you will need to acquire as soon as possible. Acknowledge that it is impossible for you to do everything at once and begin to prioritise and diarise your jobs. Make a list of everything that you need to do, arranging them in order of genuine priority. Record those tasks that need to be done immediately, in the next week, in the next month or when time allows.

You can edit what started out as an overwhelming and uncontrollable list of tasks, breaking it down into a series of smaller, more manageable ones that are spread out over a longer time period. Remember also to create buffer times to deal with unexpected and emergency tasks and to include time for your own relaxation and well-being.

Just say 'no'

Your assertiveness skills will come into play here. Much stress is caused by having too much to do and too little time in which to do it, but despite this many people still agree to take on additional responsibility. Learning to say 'no' to additional or unimportant requests can help to reduce your level of stress and may also help you develop more self-confidence.

Rest if you are unwell

If you are feeling unwell you should not carry on regardless, as your body will recover faster after you have had a short spell of rest. You have a responsibility to yourself, the people you care for and the people you work with to return to full health.

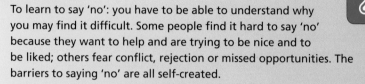

ACTIVITY 10.4

To learn to say 'no': you have to be able to understand why you may find it difficult. Some people find it hard to say 'no' because they want to help and are trying to be nice and to be liked; others fear conflict, rejection or missed opportunities. The barriers to saying 'no' are all self-created.

You might feel reluctant to respond to a request with a straight 'no', at least at first. Think instead of some pre-prepared phrases to let other people down more gently. Try practising these phrases:

- 🌡 'I am sorry but I can't commit to this as I have other priorities at the moment.'
- 🌡 'Now is not a good time as I'm in the middle of something. Why don't you ask me again at…?'
- 🌡 'I'd love to do this, but….'

Summary

The process of self-awareness is about giving you the opportunity for having clearer insights of your personality, including strengths, weaknesses, thoughts, beliefs, motivation and emotions. Self-awareness can help you to understand other people, how they see you, your attitude and how you respond to them.

It is useful to develop self-awareness as you can then make changes in the thoughts and interpretations in your mind. Self-awareness is an attribute of emotional intelligence and is an important factor in achieving success. The better you understand yourself, the better you are able to accept or change who you are. Remaining in the dark about yourself will mean that you will continue to get caught up in your own internal struggles and allow outside forces to mould and shape you.

The Johari window is a tool for self-awareness and personal development, and it helps with relationships. When you show people who you are this requires self-awareness and self-disclosure. The Johari window is essentially a lens on your own self-awareness and also a lens on self-disclosure.

Interpersonal skills are sometimes known as social skills, people skills, soft skills or life skills. They are not only about how we communicate with others, they are also associated with our confidence and our ability to listen and understand. Problem solving, decision making and personal stress management are also considered interpersonal skills. Those who have well-developed interpersonal skills are often more successful in their professional and personal lives. When you spend more effort and give more time to working, thinking and practising them then you can enhance them to their full potential.

 References

Benner, P. (1984) *From Novice to Expert. Excellence and Power in Clinical Nursing Practice.* Addison-Wesley, Menlo Park, CA

Carvalho, S., Reeves, M. and Orford, J. (2012) Relating your values, morals and ethics to nursing practice. *Independent Nurse* 20 Feb, 41

Crowell, D.M. (2011) *Complexity Leadership and Nursing's Role in Health Care Delivery.* Davis and Co, Philadelphia

Eckroth-Bucher, M. (2010) Invitation to dialogue on nursing essentials: original article self-awareness: a review and analysis of a basic nursing concept. *Advances in Nursing Science* 33(4), 297–309

Luft, J. (1970) *Group Processes: An Introduction to Group Dynamics.* Mayfield Publishing, Palo Alto, CA

Luft, J. and Ingham, H (1955) *The Johari Window: A Graphic Model of Interpersonal Awareness. Proceedings of the Western Training Laboratory in Group Development.* University of California Los Angeles, Los Angeles

Nursing and Midwifery Council (2008) *The Code: Standards of Conduct, Performance and Ethics for Nurses and Midwives.* Nursing and Midwifery Council, London

Nursing and Midwifery Council (2010) *Pre Registration Nursing Education in the UK.* http://standards.nmc-uk.org/Documents/Pre-registration%20nursing%20education%20in%20UK%20FINAL%2006092010.pdf

Royal College of Nursing (2003) *Defining Nursing.* Royal College of Nursing, London

Turton, W. (2012) Leading and managing mental health care. In Tee, S., Brown, J. and Carpenter, D. (eds), *Handbook of Mental Health Nursing.* Hodder Arnold, London, pp. 160–86

 Resources

Learn Higher

www.learnhigher.ac.uk/students.htm

A website that is committed to improving student learning by providing excellent resources to support students' learning development, packed with lots of really helpful and user-friendly resources.

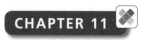
 # Terminology: Terms Used in Healthcare

WHAT THIS CHAPTER CONTAINS

- The nursing handover
- Talking the talk: language
- Anatomical landmarks
- Prefixes and suffices

Casey and Wallis (2011) make the observation that nurses and nursing staff are central to the communication process. Nurses assess, record and report on treatment and care, manage information sensitively and confidentially, deal with complaints effectively and are conscientious in reporting the things about which they are concerned.

ACTIVITY 11.1

Make a list of situations where you have been or you think you will be involved in the handing over of patient information. What do you need to consider when sharing details about a patient?

If you can accord with what Casey and Wallis (2011) have stated you need to be able to use the recognised terminology for assessing, recording and reporting on the health and well-being of the people you care for, and to participate meaningfully in patient handover to other nurses and other healthcare professionals. What must be borne in mind at all stages is that when we work with patients (and their families) their treatment and care should take into account their personal needs and preferences. Patients have the right to be fully informed and to make

The Student Nurse Toolkit: An Essential Guide for Surviving Your Course, First Edition. Ian Peate.
© 2013 John Wiley & Sons, Ltd. Published 2013 by John Wiley & Sons, Ltd.

decisions in partnership with the healthcare team. Nurses and other members of the healthcare team should provide the patient with information that they can understand and that is relevant to their circumstances. At all times nurses should treat the patient with respect, sensitivity and understanding and provide explanations simply and clearly.

The nursing handover

Intentional rounding

Following a number of critical reports, concern has been expressed about the need to ensure that essential aspects of nursing care are consistently delivered. In January 2011 the Prime Minister called for changes in the way that nurses delivered care. One the various recommendations was for NHS hospitals to implement hourly nursing rounds, checking that the fundamental needs of patients were being met. This approach was related to what is known in the USA as 'intentional rounding'; in the UK a similar approach is known as 'care rounds'. This edict was met with much discussion in the general and nursing media.

The key elements of intentional rounding in acute care, described by the Studer Group (2007) and Bartley (2011), are the four 'Ps':

1 **P**ositioning: making sure the patient is comfortable and assessing the risk of pressure ulcers,
2 **P**ersonal needs: scheduling patient trips to the bathroom to avoid risk of falls,
3 **P**ain: asking patients to describe their pain level on a scale of 0–10,
4 **P**lacement: making sure the items a patient needs are within easy reach.

Halm (2009) suggests that during each round the nurse should undertake the following:

- use an opening phrase to introduce yourself and put the patient at ease, perform scheduled tasks and ask about the four Ps (see above),
- assess the care environment (e.g. fall hazards, temperature of the room),
- use closing key words, such as 'is there anything else I can do for you before I go?', and explain when the patient will be checked again,
- document the round.

Not all hospitals in the UK have implemented intentional rounding. Where intentional rounding has been introduced, the method varies (National Nursing Research Unit, 2012). The focus has been on registered nurses undertaking rounds; student nurses and healthcare assistants also participate. There are some hospitals where registered nurses, student nurses and healthcare assistants may undertake rounds alternately each hour and in some places the whole interdisciplinary team is involved.

The frequency of rounds between hospitals and wards also varies. Patients who are acutely ill, people with intensive mental health needs and those with dementia may benefit from more frequent checks. It is usual for rounds to be undertaken every hour or 2 hours throughout the day and night depending on the patient's clinical condition or their level of need. There is also variation associated with which patients to include. In certain hospitals, only those patients who have been deemed at risk of falling or having skin damage, or those requiring emergency or critical care, are included (Halm, 2009).

Types of handover

Handover of patients does not only occur in hospitals. The nurse may be required to provide handover of care (a narrative about the patient) or even transfer the care of the patient to another health or social care agency. The practice nurse may need to hand over details about the patient to the community nurse, the night site coordinator may need to brief the medical team about a patient's intensive care transfer needs to another specialist hospital or the children's nurse may need to handover the care of a child to social care agencies. The most important thing about handover is to communicate effectively.

There are many places where handover can occur. The most obvious one is usually at the nurse's station or the ward office and then at the patient's bedside at the end and beginning of a shift. These venues change, however, depending on the environment in which the patient is being nursed; for example, in places of detention this may occur in a secure prison setting.

The ward handover

At the change of nursing shifts handover is the communication between two shifts of nurses where the specific purpose is to communicate information about patients under their care. The overall objective of the handover is to ensure that patient care continues seamlessly and safely, providing the oncoming nursing staff with relevant information to begin care provision immediately. The principles of confidentiality must apply during all stages of handover.

Handover style appears to depend very much upon local circumstances. There are a variety of methods that are used to undertake handover, and some healthcare providers have formalised these methods with the aim of providing consistency.

ACTIVITY 11.2

When you are next on a practice placement (wherever that may be) seek out the guidelines or policy that has been written to guide nurses when undertaking handover.

Some care areas use preprinted computerised patient handover sheets, which allow the nurses to concentrate on the verbal handover being given. At the end of each shift the handover sheets are shredded. Pothier *et al.* (2005) suggest that the nursing handover process should be considered as a critical aspect of providing quality care in contemporary healthcare environments. In addition, the quality of a report given can potentially delay an individual nurse's ability to provide care for up to 1–2 hours.

Handover varies in length. A 'full report' can last between 30 minutes, an hour or longer, whereas a report with the 'headlines' may give a quick overall patient update following a particularly busy part of the day or after a specific incident (see above and intentional rounding).

There are a number of styles of handing over:

- ☥ verbal handover,
- ☥ tape-recorded handover,
- ☥ bedside handover,
- ☥ written handover.

No single style is more superior to any other. Circumstances may vary from one area to another in relation to numbers of patients, dependency and staffing levels, and these factors can influence the style used. Often an eclectic approach is used, mixing and matching the various styles. Handover should not just be directed towards the nurse in charge. All nurses starting a shift need a handover.

PEARLS OF WISDOM

Always ensure you arrive on time for handover. Arriving late is unprofessional; it can disrupt the important act of communicating care needs. It may be an idea to have two pens with you – a black one and red one – so that you are able to highlight things that are important. Use red as a prompt.

Often a safety briefing is undertaken at the beginning of a shift. Lasting only 2–3 minutes, the focus is on specific patient safety issues for that clinical area on that shift. Currie (2002) suggests using the mnemonic CUBAN to set a quality standard for each verbal handover, as follows.

Confidential: be sure that information cannot be overheard. Notes must remain with you all the time, must not be taken out of the clinical area and must not become part of the patient's case notes or part of any assignment you are doing.

Uninterrupted: find a quiet area where there are no distractions. Commence on time, at the beginning of the shift.

Brief: keep information relevant; too much information can be confusing. Do not pass on unnecessary or unethical information. Do not label or stereotype.

Accurate: all information must be correct and ensure that no patients are missed out. Care plans should be up to date at the beginning and the end of every shift. Information should be clear and concise without the use of jargon.

Named nurse: the person who has looked after the patient should give the handover. This enhances continuity.

There will be many demands placed on you during your working day. When working with your mentor or another member of the ward team you will need to triage what needs to be done first and what can safely be left until later. You cannot do it all at once. It will take you time to learn how to organise what absolutely needs to be done, what is important, what can wait and what you need not to worry about if it does not get done: this is called experience.

Box 11.1 provides you with tips to help you when you are taking part in a handover.

Box 11.1 Tips that may help when taking handover

Using a structured approach will help you avoid information overload and let you focus on what is relevant. The following five points may help when listening to the report.
1. Patient's name, diagnosis, doctor and past relevant history
2. Patient's date of admission, reason for admission and/or date of operation
3. Present restrictions? For example, nil by mouth, fluids only, diabetic diet, non-weight-bearing
4. Plan of care; for example, the patient's main problem/need is…and he/she will need…. The next problem/need is…and will need…and so on.
5. What part you can play in the next shift? The handover should show progression: what needs to happen during the next shift.

SECTION SUMMARY

Handover takes place at a number of locations and the way this happens is dependent on the nursing environment. Intentional rounding takes many different forms: it can result in positive patient outcomes. Further evaluation of intentional rounding is needed to determine the evidence for its effectiveness.

Written handovers may prove to be more accurate and a much less time-consuming method than other methods. However, verbal handovers remain the most popular way of communication during shift reporting. This method can be enhanced with a pre-prepared handover sheet and can avoid the loss of essential information that may result after serious patient incidents.

Talking the talk: the language

> On my first practice placement I was with the practice nurse and I attended a practice meeting where we were discussing a group of patients. I thought my head would explode with all of the words they were using. I said to my mentor, it's like they are speaking a foreign language, she said, 'they are: it's Greek'. So I went to uni to learn nursing and also came out with an understanding of Latin and Greek. *Cynthia, third year student*

One of the skills the nurse needs to develop is to be able to decipher and understand the meaning of new words and a dictionary full of abbreviations. Learning to talk the talk is important and so is understanding the language (it is one of the tools of the trade), but using jargon to impress is not impressive. Jargon, nursing or otherwise, should never be used in front of patients and their families, as it can scare and alienate them.

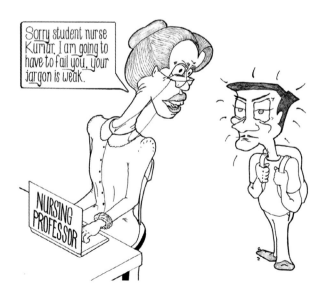

ACTIVITY 11.3

Imagine how a patient would feel if we spoke to them in the same way as we speak to our colleagues or fellow healthcare professionals, using the language of nursing. How might they feel hearing or reading this?

> Mrs Upton, NBM from 0830h for a CABG at 1400h. To be given stat clexine and then QDS antibiotic as Rx. Needs CXR, ECG, FBC and ABGs. Drip and suck NGT PRN. C/O left iliac pain SpR informed.

While you are attending your practice placements and when you are in university you will come across words, abbreviations, diseases and conditions that you may have never heard of before. There are hundreds of terms to learn.

Abbreviations and acronyms

You will use many such terms and abbreviations when writing and reading patient notes, completing care planning, writing reports and working on university assignments. The use of abbreviations in nursing and medicine is widespread. It is usual for each department or ward or community care setting to have their own list of accepted abbreviations. In those areas where such a list has not been produced, there is a danger that staff will use a great number of different abbreviations, which are accepted but can possibly mean something else to each member of the team. Dimond (2011) suggests that these lists should be reviewed regularly. The upshot of this is confusion and there is a real possibility that patients can be harmed by the misunderstandings that may ensue.

PEARLS OF WISDOM

When working with other healthcare professionals you may have to use jargon but whenever you are unsure – about either the words being used or the multitude of abbreviations – you must seek clarification. Don't muddle through.

The NMC's position on abbreviations is that records should not include unnecessary abbreviations (Nursing and Midwifery Council, 2010). Nearly all abbreviations have multiple different possible expansions. It is usually easy to disambiguate (that is, remove uncertainty of the meanings) an abbreviation that has alternative meanings.

You can distinguish AKA ('above-knee amputation') from AKA ('also known as') by the context of the sentence, which can often help determine the meaning.

A number of everyday nursing and medical abbreviations are used appropriately and safely; for example, BP for blood pressure. If this kind of abbreviation had to be written in full each time it was used it would add considerably to the time needed to complete records. However, there are dangers associated with the use of abbreviations. PT could mean patient, physiotherapist, part time or prothrombin; BID might mean twice daily or brought in dead.

Berman (2007) suggests that there are many abbreviations that cannot easily be disambiguated, even by experts in a knowledge domain, where another, very similar, term with the same abbreviation is mistakenly used.

Abbreviations that cannot always be disambiguated are particularly dangerous and are a potential source of nursing and medical errors. There are some examples in Table 11.1.

Table 11.1 Some abbreviations and their possible meaning

Abbreviation	Possible meaning
ABG	Arterial blood gases, aortic bifurcation graft or aortobifemoral graft
AHA	Acquired haemolytic anaemia or autoimmune haemolytic anaemia
ASCVD	Arteriosclerotic cardiovascular disease or arteriosclerotic cerebrovascular disease
CHD	Congenital heart disease, congestive heart disease or coronary heart disease
DOA	Date of admission or dead on arrival
FBC	Full blood count or fluid balance chart
HZO	Herpes zoster ophthalmicus or herpes zoster oticus
IBD	Inflammatory bowel disease or irritable bowel disease
LLL	Left lower lid, left lower lip, left lower lobe or left lower lung
MS	Multiple sclerosis or mitral stenosis
MVR	Mitral valve regurgitation, mitral valve repair or mitral valve replacement
NKDA	No known drug allergies or nonketotic diabetic acidosis
PE	Pulmonary effusion, pulmonary embolectomy or pulmonary embolism
PID	Pelvic inflammatory disease or prolapsed intervertebral disc

An acronym is an abbreviation formed from the initial letters of a set of words and pronounced as a word. Just as confusion may arise when using abbreviations, the same is true of acronyms.

Anatomical landmarks

Some terms that are used are based on the human body. Terms that are associated with certain sections of the body are called descriptive terms. All references to the body are made in relation to the anatomical position (see Figure 11.1), which refers to the standing forward-facing body. An imaginary line is drawn down the centre from head to feet, dividing the body into two equal halves. When we read the word medial it refers to a part that is closer to the midline/centre; lateral means further from the midline/centre.

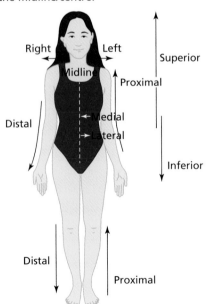

Figure 11.1 Anatomical planes (i).

Imagine that another line has been drawn, this one dividing the upper and lower body into two halves (see Figure 11.2). The line is right under the navel. The term superior in anatomical positioning refers to above that line and inferior means below the line. Turn the body to face sideways (as in Figure 11.2). Draw an imaginary line down the centre. The term anterior (ventral is sometimes used) means towards the front. The term posterior (or dorsal) means towards the back.

The abdomen also has anatomical landmarks and is divided into four sections, known as quadrants. The quadrants are shown on Figure 11.3 and the landmarks are listed in Table 11.2.

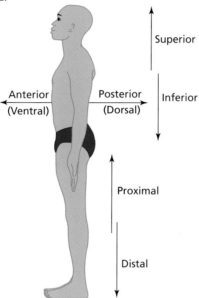

Figure 11.2 Anatomical planes (ii).

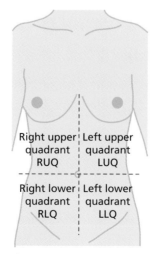

Figure 11.3 The abdominal quadrants.

Table 11.2 Abdominal anatomical landmarks

Position	Term	Abdominal contents
Right upper quadrant	RUQ	Right lobe of liver, gall bladder, duodenum, head of pancreas, right adrenal gland, upper lobe of right kidney, section of ascending colon, section of transverse colon
Right lower quadrant	RLQ	Caecum, appendix, section of ascending colon, right ovary, right fallopian tube, right ureter, right spermatic cord, part of uterus
Left upper quadrant	LUQ	Left lobe of liver, stomach, spleen, upper lobe of left kidney, pancreas, left adrenal gland, splenic flexure of the colon, section of transverse colon, section of descending colon
Left lower quadrant	LLQ	Lower lobe of left kidney, sigmoid colon, section of descending colon, left ovary, left fallopian tube, left ureter, left spermatic cord, part of uterus

The abdomen can also be divided into nine other regions:

1 umbilical
2 epigastric
3 hypogastric
4 left lumbar
5 right lumbar
6 left iliac
7 right iliac
8 left hypochondriac
9 right hypochondriac

Prefixes and suffixes

There are many other forms of medical jargon that you will have to decipher. An understanding of word roots, prefixes and suffixes can help you work out the words that you see and will use when you become more competent and confident.

A word root is the foundation of a medical term. Word roots usually (but not always) refer to the body part being described. Most of the words are derived from Greek or Latin, and you should also take note that the American English spelling of the words can sometimes be different. A prefix is added to the beginning of a word to change or add to its meaning. A suffix can also be added to the end of a word, also changing its meaning. Table 11.3 provides some examples of word roots and their meanings, Table 11.4 details some common prefixes along with their meanings and examples, and Table 11.5 considers the use of suffixes.

Table 11.3 Some word roots and their meanings

Word root	Meaning
aden	gland
broncho	bronchi
chol	gall bladder
craino	skull
dent	teeth
haemo	blood
hepato	liver
hystero	uterus
myo	muscle
nephro	kidney
pulmo	lung
uro	urine

Table 11.4 Some prefixes, their meanings and examples

Prefix	Meaning	Example	Meaning
a...	without	afebrile	Without fever
brady...	slow	bradycardia	Slow pulse rate
dys...	pain or difficulty	dysuria	Painful urination
hyper...	above or excessive	hypertension	High blood pressure
hypo...	below or deficient	hypothermia	Low body temperature
peri...	around	periorbital	Around the eye
poly...	many	polyuria	Passing large amounts of urine
post...	after	post-menopausal	After the menopause
pre...	before	prepubertal	Before puberty
tachy...	fast	tachycardia	Fast pulse rate

Table 11.5 Examples of suffixes and their meanings

Suffix	Meaning
...aemia	blood (anaemia)
...ectomy	removal of (splenectomy)
...gram	record (electroencephalogram)
...itis	inflammation (appendicitis)
...logy	study of (cytology)
...oma	tumour (seminoma)
...otomy	incision (tracheotomy)
...plegia	paralysis (tetraplegia)
...pnoea	respirations (dyspnoea)

ACTIVITY 11.4

What do the following words mean?

Word	Meaning
splenectomy	
appendicitis	
electroencephalogram	
anaemia	
cytology	
seminoma	
tracheotomy	
tetraplegia	
dyspnoea	

Mnemonics

Mnemonics are devices, such as a pattern of letters, ideas or associations, that assist in remembering something. They can also be fun to use and they are often used in anatomy. See Table 11.6.

Table 11.6 Examples of some mnemonics

Fact	Mnemonic
Remember the basic framework of the Glasgow Coma Scale	**Eye opening:** 4 eyes (glasses) **Motor:** 6 cylinder engine **Verbal:** Jackson 5
A proven myocardial infarction should be met by MONA	**M** = morphine **O** = oxygen **N** = nitrates **A** = aspirin
Causes of haematuria	Use the mnemonic SITTT as an aid in evaluating the cause of haematuria: **S** = stone **I** = infection **T** = trauma **T** = tumour **T** = tuberculosis
For remembering the order of the cranial nerves	Oh Oh Oh! To Touch And Feel Very Good Velvet, Absolute Happiness! **O**lfactory, **O**ptic, **O**culomotor, **T**rochlear, **T**rigeminal, **A**bducens, **F**acial, **V**estibulocochlear, **G**lossopharyngeal, **V**agus, **A**ccessory, **H**ypoglossal
The principles of treatment in soft tissue injuries, especially muscular injuries	RICE **R** = rest **I** = ice **C** = compression **E** = elevation

Summary

In communicating with other healthcare professionals, for example when attending patient handover, you will be using words, reading reports and speaking with other healthcare professionals in a language that may be new to you. This language, the jargon used or the technical terminology can be learned and you can then talk the talk. There are many terms, abbreviations, conditions and diseases that you will need to learn about. One way of getting to grips with this is to understand roots, prefixes and suffixes. Lots of the words used are derived from Greek and Latin, so you are not only learning how to nurse you are also learning a new language.

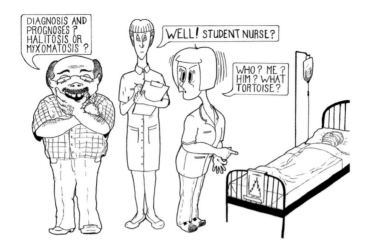

Anatomical landmarks can be complex, but once you have mastered them your confidence in discussing patient care with others will soar as you learn new words and phrases and you understand what anatomical aspects are being discussed.

It is unacceptable to use jargon and technical terminology in front of and with a patient and their family. It can cause them undue stress and anxiety. Just think how you felt when you first heard healthcare professionals discussing patients: you may have felt totally out of your depth, ignorant, sacred and overwhelmed.

 ## References

Bartley, A. (2011) *The Hospital Pathways Project. Making it Happen: Intentional Rounding.* The King's Fund Point of Care and The Health Foundation, London

Berman, J.J. (2007) *Biomedical Infomatics.* Johns and Bartlett, New York

Casey, A. and Wallis, A (2011) Effective communication: principle of nursing practice E. *Nursing Standard* 25(32), 35–7

Currie, J. (2002) Improving the efficiency of patient handover. *Emergency Nurse* 10(3), 24–7

Dimond, B. (2011) *Legal Aspects of Nursing*, 6th edn. Pearson, Harlow

Halm, M. (2009) Hourly rounds: what does the evidence indicate? *American Association of Critical Care Nurses* 18, 581–4

National Nursing Research Unit (2012) *Intentional Rounding: What is the Evidence?* www.kcl .ac.uk/nursing/research/nnru/Policy/Currentissue/Policy-Plus-Issue35.pdf

Nursing and Midwifery Council (2010) *Record keeping, Guidance for Nurses and Midwives.* Nursing and Midwifery Council, London

Pothier, D., Monteiro, P., Mookitiar, M. and Shaw, M. (2005) Pilot study to show the loss of important data in nursing handover. *British Journal of Nursing* 14(20), 1090–3

Studer Group (2007) *Best Practices: Sacred Heart Hospital, Pensacola, Florida. Hourly Rounding Supplement.* Studer Group, FL

Resources

National Nursing Research Unit

www.kcl.ac.uk/nursing/research/nnru/index.aspx

The NNRU is based at King's College London and undertakes high-quality research and reviews that inform policy and practice relevant to the nursing workforce.

Plain English Campaign

www.plainenglish.co.uk/

The Plain English Campaign has been campaigning against gobbledygook, jargon and misleading public information. Its aim is for everyone to have access to clear and concise information.

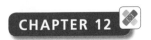
Evidence-Based Practice

WHAT THIS CHAPTER CONTAINS

- What is evidence-based practice?
- Evidence practice and research
- Sources of evidence
- How to access the sources
- Barriers to undertaking and implementing evidence-based practice

You may have heard nurses and academic staff on placement and in the university refer to the evidence base for practice. The NMC (Nursing and Midwifery Council, 2008) requires nurses, as autonomous practitioners, to deliver essential care to a very high standard and to provide complex care using the best available evidence and technology where appropriate. The NMC standards for pre-registration education (Nursing and Midwifery Council, 2010) demand that students develop practice, and promote and sustain change.

As a graduate nurse you must demonstrate throughout your programme that you can think analytically, and use problem-solving approaches to care and evidence in decision making, keep up with technical advances and meet future expectations. The care that you provide must be based on research, underpinned by a sound evidence base. You are also required to employ critical thinking when responding effectively to the needs of people.

The programme you are undertaking recognises that as an adult you will bring with you a range of qualities, including not only expertise in your subject but also the ability to manage your own learning. Part of this is making use of sources of evidence to make judgements, which is fundamental to twenty-first century nursing. Hence the use of evidence is central to your studies and your practice.

The Student Nurse Toolkit: An Essential Guide for Surviving Your Course, First Edition. Ian Peate.
© 2013 John Wiley & Sons, Ltd. Published 2013 by John Wiley & Sons, Ltd.

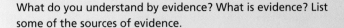

What do you understand by evidence? What is evidence? List some of the sources of evidence.

Evidence-based practice

We are being required more and more to base our practice on sound evidence. This is absolutely correct. It is becoming increasingly necessary for us to support any clinical decisions we make with a rationale. We have to justify our actions, not only in an ethical and moral way as laid down in our code of conduct (Nursing and Midwifery Council, 2008), but also in the treatments that we offer to people.

In searching for the best possible outcomes for patients we must engage in research to determine how we can achieve those outcomes (Newell and Burnard, 2011). Areas that may be subjected to study and investigation are wide and varied. Examples include illness and recovery trajectories, how care is managed and organised and the impact of dementia on a person's ability to express pain.

When care provision (whatever this may be) lacks an evidence base then there is potential to do harm. When nurses use and implement evidence-based practice (EBP) they are adding value to the patient experience and can legitimately provide evidence underpinning their actions. However, they must have a sound foundation in what EBP is and how it can be used in practice to provide evidence-based care. Defining EBP is therefore essential.

 We had done a module at uni about EBP and one of the assessments was to identify where EBP was being used in the clinical areas. I was shocked that many of the staff I worked with had no idea about EBP. My mentor was brilliant: she and I learned together, taking turns to find the answers. We ended up like detectives. *Shola, third year student nurse*

Defining evidence-based practice

Sears (2006) suggests that EBP is a process that enables nurses to make clinical decisions using the best available evidence, along with their own clinical experiences, including patient preferences. Evidence-based medicine was a term coined by Sackett (1994) and since then has been used far and wide. Sackett *et al.* (1996) define evidence-based practice as:

> ...the conscious, explicit, and judicious use of current best evidence in making decisions about the care of individual patients.

The definition is often extended to other fields of practice where practitioners are required to make decisions about people and of groups of people concerning their care. As such, EBP has been extended to nursing.

Straus *et al.* (2011) suggest that evidence-based medicine necessitates a combination of the best research evidence with clinical expertise as well as the patient's unique values and circumstances. EBP and evidence-based medicine are more than just about evidence alone: they include and embrace the individual experience. The nurse–patient relationship means that this is a complex process and that the underlying aim is to do the right thing for the patient.

'Research' in the definition of Straus *et al.* (2011) concerns research that is clinically relevant with a patient focus, associated with efficacy and safer therapeutic, rehabilitative and preventative strategies. The ability to use clinical skills and past experience is implemented to quickly identify any risks to the patient and any problems that they may have. It also involves ensuring a patient's personal values and expectations are taken into account; for example, their unique preferences, concerns and expectations. This definition considers not only the scientific perspective but also expertise and the individual's preferences.

There are critics of EBP. O'Halloran (2010) suggests that nurses should neither abandon EBP nor accept it uncritically. Considering cost-effectiveness in EBP may lead some to suggest that it can result in cost cutting or treatment rationing. EBP has the ability to cut costs without having negative patient outcomes; for example, efforts to reduce the number and severity of falls and pressure ulcers. By implementing evidence-based guidelines about falls and pressure ulcers, care can be improved and the number and severity of adverse outcomes can decrease. Failure to use evidence according to Berwick (2003) results in care that is of lower quality, less effective and more expensive.

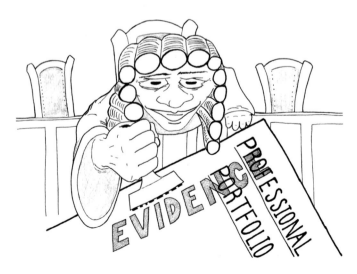

EBP is central to nursing practice because:

- it helps to provide care that meets the needs of the individual,
- it results in improved patient outcomes and patient satisfaction,
- it adds to the science of nursing,
- it ensures that practice is current and relevant,
- it enhances confidence in decision making, making it more explicit,
- it informs policies and procedures, ensuring they are current and include the latest research.

SECTION SUMMARY

All nurses should be striving to provide care that is underpinned by a sound evidence base; this can enable nurses to justify their actions. Care that has no evidence base can cause harm.
There are many positive patient outcomes associated with care that has an evidence base. The patient is at the heart of everything that the nurse does when such an approach is utilised.

EBP is all about using the best evidence for the effective care of individuals, using it with the person's best interests in mind. Nurses must strive to provide the best quality of care that they can, drawing upon the available evidence.

Evidence-based practice and research

Research may not have all of the answers to questions raised in association with care delivery, and where this is lacking there are other forms of evidence that may be equally informative. EBP is wider than research-based practice. It encompasses a number of other forms of knowing, such as (and not limited to) those described by Carper in the late 1970s (Carper, 1978):

- empirical evidence (the science of nursing),
- aesthetic evidence (the art of nursing),
- ethical evidence (the moral component),
- personal evidence.

Newell and Burnard (2011) suggest that the trend towards evidence-based care is an attempt to put information at the heart of healthcare and make it usable to nurses and others.

The terms research and EBP are often used together. Indeed, many textbooks have both words in their title and this is done for a reason: the evidence base and research process are very closely aligned. The nurse must have an understanding and appreciation of the fundamental concepts associated with the various research methods and the research process as this is the grounding for using research evidence in the delivery of care as well as participating in EBP in the workplace.

The research process and an evidence-based approach are both systematic, but their purposes are different. Using an EBP approach the nurse needs to consider the available research findings, results that point to quality improvement and other forms of evaluation data, audit and expert opinion with the intention of identifying methods of improvement.

Nurses carry out a number of roles with the aim of ensuring and providing EBP and they must constantly ask questions, such as, 'What is the evidence for this intervention?' or 'How do we provide best practice?' and 'Are these the highest achievable outcomes for the patient, their family and nurses?' EBP confronts nurses by asking them to consider the what, how and why behind current methods and processes, encouraging them to search for improvement. It challenges the rote, traditional approaches used in care provision that are so often based on heresay, or 'this is the way we have always done it', or care that is based on traditions, myths, suppositions or outdated textbooks. Practice-based knowledge does not translate into quality patient care or health outcomes. EBP provides a critical strategy ensuring that your care is up to date and that it mirrors the latest research evidence. EBP may have opinion, for example expert opinion, that is an integral aspect of that practice. EBP is not research utilisation, quality improvement nor nursing research, although it may be related to each of these processes.

In contrast, the aim of research is to generate new knowledge about a phenomenon or to validate current knowledge. Nursing research involves systematic enquiry, particularly designed to develop, refine and extend nursing knowledge. It is a structured method of measuring and evaluating outcomes of various procedures, practices and hypotheses. Any new findings that arise can be integrated into everyday nursing practice. This is then referred to as EBP. The evidence in EBP is the result of research: nursing practice is based on this evidence. Greenberg and Pyle (2004) suggest that EBP, in its broadest sense, is the use of evidence to support decision making in healthcare. An EBP project can very easily lead to a research study or quality-improvement initiative. Table 12.1 outlines the differences between research and EBP.

Table 12.1 Differences between evidence-based practice and research

Research	Evidence-based practice
Systematic and deliberate investigation	Systematic search for, as well as an appraisal of, the best available evidence
Problem to be investigated clearly specified	Using the evidence to make clinical decisions, the research usually provides the evidence
Statement of predetermined outcome (i.e. results and recommendations)	The needs of the individual patient are taken into account as well as the research evidence base
Contributes to understanding (for example, the body of knowledge that informs nursing)	Results in a change in practice

Source: adapted from Carnwell (2001).

The evidence base cycle

According to Newell and Burnard (2011) EBP can be broken down into five stages, as shown in Box 12.1. EBP always begins and ends with the patient.

Box 12.1 The five stages of the evidence-based cycle

1 Asking answerable questions: this recognises that there is a need for new information and this information need has to be converted into an answerable question. PICO is a mnemonic used to help remember the key components of a well-focused question (see below). The question has to identify the key problem of the patient, what treatment/intervention is being considered for the patient, what alternative treatment/intervention is being considered (if any) and what is the outcome that is desired or to be avoided or promoted:

   P = patient problem,
   I = intervention,
   C = comparison (if any),
   O = outcome.

2 Finding the best available evidence: this requires a search for the right evidence. There are many databases that can be used to search for evidence. These include CINAHL (Cumulative Index to Nursing and Allied Health Literature; a database of references to journals and papers, focusing on nursing and midwifery journals, that includes primary journals for allied health professionals), MEDLINE (a database containing journal citations and abstracts for biomedical literature from around the world) or databases within the Cochrane library (an online database of high-quality evidence to inform healthcare decision making). Being able to input the correct terms or phrases into the various databases is a skill that must be honed. Other sources are available that can provide best evidence. For example, PRODIGY is a reliable source of evidence-based information and practical 'know how' about common conditions managed in primary and first-contact care. Organisations such as Scottish Intercollegiate Guidelines Network (SIGN) and National Institute for Health and Care Excellence (NICE) produce guidelines with the evidence that was used to inform.

3 Appraising the evidence for its validity and applicability: at this stage the evidence gathered is critically appraised to establish its validity and potential usefulness. When the evidence has been found that will answer the question the next stage is to critically appraise it to determine whether it is valid. This will involve asking the following questions.

   - Can the evidence or results of the research study be trusted: have they been formed through an appropriate methodology during the research process?
   - What is the evidence saying and what does it mean?
   - Does the research/evidence answer your question?
   - Is it all relevant to your clinical practice?

4 Applying the results to clinical practice: incorporating the evidence into clinical practice, being aware of the benefits and risks of implementing any changes and also being mindful of the benefits and risks of excluding any alternatives.

5 Evaluation and reflecting on the performance of the EBP: this stage is essential to decide whether the action taken has achieved the desired results.

EBP, like the nursing process, is a continuous process: it is dynamic and cyclical (see Figure 12.1).

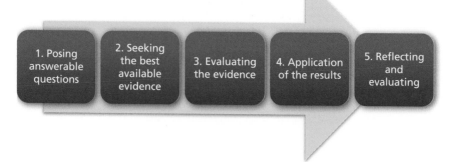

1. Posing answerable questions

2. Seeking the best available evidence

3. Evaluating the evidence

4. Application of the results

5. Reflecting and evaluating

Figure 12.1 The stages associated with evidence-based practice. *Source*: data from Newell and Burnard (2011).

 ## The evidence base

Evidence, according to Rycroft-Malone *et al.* (2004), is more than findings from formal research projects. These authors go on to suggest that there are four distinct sources of evidence:

1 research,
2 clinical or professional experience,
3 patients and their carers,
4 the local context in which you practice (including audit and evaluation data, local professional networks and feedback from quality assurance programmes).

Nurses need to know where to find the evidence, what to do with it once it has been located and how to apply it. Drawing upon all of the resources above can help to ensure the effective use of evidence in care provision.

The evidence used must be the most up to date and relevant. Research findings may not always be the best source of evidence in some cases, as there are some areas where research has not been carried out. There may be instances where research has been done, but the data generated are not relevant for the particular situation that you find yourself in or the person you are providing care to. In some situations the next best option may be evidence from personal experience and from discussions with other healthcare professionals, such as a physiotherapist.

SECTION SUMMARY

Research and EBP are terms that are often used interchangeably. EBP can be broken down into five stages: (1) the question, (2) finding the evidence, (3) appraising the evidence, (4) acting on the evidence and (5) evaluating the process and reflecting upon it. It is a continual, cyclical process.

There are four sources of evidence in healthcare: research, clinical or professional experience, patients and their carers, and the local context in which the nurse practices, such as internal audits, local professional networks and feedback from quality assurance programmes.

Hierarchies of evidence

A hierarchy of evidence exists, which ranks the types of evidence in terms of quality. In 1979 the Canadian Task Force on the Periodic Health Examination published one of the first efforts to explicitly characterise the level of evidence underlying healthcare recommendations and the strength of recommendations (*Canadian Medical Association Journal*, 1979).

Clinical decisions should be based on the highest-ranking forms of evidence as well as from all other sources and ranks. A commonly used aid to assess the worth of the material found is the hierarchy of evidence; this is also used in clinical decision making. The hierarchy permits research-based evidence to be graded according to its design. It is ranked in order of decreasing internal validity indicating the confidence that decision and policy makers can have in the findings. Petticrew and Roberts (2003) note that the hierarchy of evidence remains a source of debate, as the term is contentious when applied to health promotion and public health. Table 12.2 provides an example of a grading system that outlines the levels of a hierarchy. Table 12.3 outlines the levels of evidence as described by Muir Gray (1997).

Table 12.2 A hierarchy of evidence

Rank	Methodology	Description
1	Systematic review and meta-analysis	Systematic review: review of a body of data that uses explicit methods to locate primary studies and precise criteria to assess and evaluate their quality. Meta-analysis: a statistical analysis combining or integrating the results of a number of independent clinical trials that are considered by the analyst to be 'combinable'; this is usually to the level of re-analysing the original data; sometimes called pooling or quantitative synthesis. Systematic review and meta-analysis are sometimes known as 'overviews'.

Table 12.2 *(continued)*

Rank	Methodology	Description
2	Randomised controlled trial	Individuals are randomly allocated to a control group and a group that receive an explicit intervention. Other than this the two groups are identical for any significant variables and are followed up for specific end points.
3	Cohort study	Groups are selected on the basis of their exposure to a specific agent and are followed-up for specific outcomes.
4	Case-controlled study	A study comparing two groups of people: those with the disease or condition under study (cases) and a very similar group of people who have not got the disease or condition (controls).
5	Cross-sectional survey	A survey or interview of a sample of the population of interest at a single point in time.
6	Case report	A report based on one single patient or subject, occasionally collected together into a short series.
7	Expert opinion	A consensus of experience from the good and the great: expert committees and respected authorities.
8	Anecdotal	Something that a friend may have told you after a meeting.

Source: data from Mantzoukas (2007), Larrabee (2009) and Jolley (2010).

Table 12.3 Levels of evidence

Level	Description
1	Robust evidence from at least one systematic review
2	Robust evidence from at least one randomised controlled trail of appropriate size
3	Evidence from well-designed non-randomised trails
4	Evidence from well-designed non-experimental studies from more than one research group or centre
5	Expert authority opinion or reports of experts

Source: adapted from Muir Gray (1997).

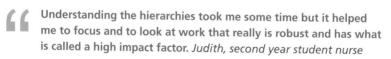

" Understanding the hierarchies took me some time but it helped me to focus and to look at work that really is robust and has what is called a high impact factor. *Judith, second year student nurse*

SECTION SUMMARY

A hierarchy of evidence ranks the different types of evidence in terms of quality. This is not set in stone and there is much debate about the ranking of some forms of evidence; for example, qualitative evidence. Any clinical decision should not only be based on the highest ranking forms of evidence but it should also draw on all sources and ranks of evidence.

ACTIVITY 12.2

What is ranked first in the hierarchy of evidence? What is ranked last in the hierarchy of evidence?

 ## Accessing the evidence

When the question has been decided upon (see stage 1 of the evidence-based cycle; Box 12.1) the evidence has to be accessed in order for it to be appraised (stage 3).

PEARLS OF WISDOM

Constructing a well-built clinical question can lead directly to a well-built search strategy.

When undertaking EBP you have to be able to search the primary literature to find answers to the clinical question posed. There are millions of published reports, journal articles, correspondences and studies available for you to choose from. Picking the best resource to search is an important decision. There are a number of large databases available (some of these have been discussed already, such as CINAHL and MEDLINE) that provide access to the primary literature. Other sources (secondary sources) – for example, clinical evidence – will provide an assessment of the original study. The Cochrane Library offers access to systematic reviews that summarise the results from various studies.

It is essential that you understand how to use the electronic resources available at the library in your university or the various learning resources at your workplace.

Sources available include the following:

- peer-reviewed journals are journals which include research-based articles in their publication range; research-based articles usually provide enough details about the methodology used for the reader to make an informed judgement about the study's validity and the clinical relevance of the findings; some journals also have an impact factor;
- government publications; for example, funded research reports, discussion papers, conference proceedings, government policies and enquiry outcomes;
- information produced by organisations and professional bodies such as the RCN; these are often free and offer further sources of evidence;
- indexes and abstracts to theses;
- reference collections; for example, specific dictionaries and encyclopaedias;
- proceedings from conferences;
- information produced by pharmaceutical companies;
- discussion and networking groups;
- newspapers.

Depending on the question you have set and are trying to answer there may be so much information available that you feel overwhelmed by it all. To avoid this you will need to narrow your search with the aim of obtaining a manageable number of articles.

ACTIVITY 12.3

In your university library, seek out the subject librarian for health and human sciences. Spend some time with him or her and look at the numerous databases you may be required to access when looking at or devising care that has an evidence base.

You should view this section of the chapter only as a taster: searching the literature effectively requires much skill and here the principles of searching the research literature are outlined. Figure 12.2 offers further guidance on searching the literature.

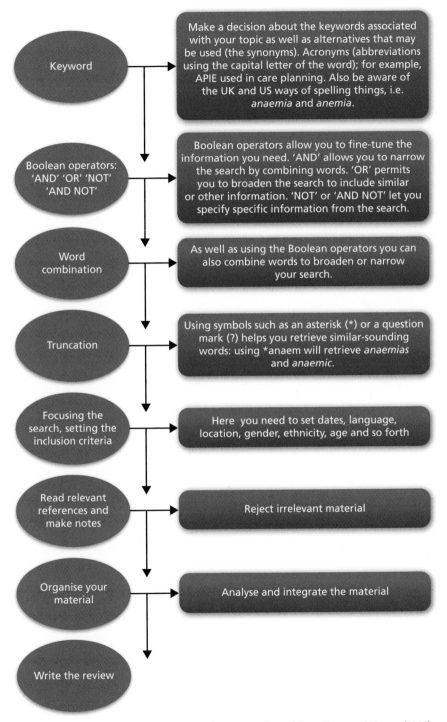

Figure 12.2 The steps in the literature search. *Source*: adapted from Burns and Groves (2011) and Polit and Beck (2011).

Carrying out a literature search can be a lengthy and complex process; however, the time taken is well worth the investment. You must be focused, organised and systematic in your approach, ensuring that you keep detailed records of the searches you have made as well as the information you have retrieved. Enlist the help of the subject librarian, who will be able to provide you with assistance from their expert perspective.

Inclusion criteria

Inclusion criteria are characteristics that are key to the problem under scrutiny. Sometimes these are referred to as eligibility criteria, meaning that the sample population must possess the named characteristics. Examples of inclusion or eligibility criteria include:

- appropriate age groups,
- language, for example English,
- location or geography,
- time period, for example between 2000 and 2013.

The inclusion criterion will mean that the results of the search will be limited to articles reviewed in databases such as Health Technology Assessment (HTA), Cochrane Database of Systematic Reviews (CDSR) and Databases of Abstracts of Reviews of Effectiveness (DARE). DARE complements the CDSR by providing a selection of quality-assessed reviews in those subjects for which there is currently no Cochrane review (Burns and Grove, 2011; Hurley *et al.*, 2011).

Exclusion criteria

Just as there are inclusion criteria there may also be exclusion criteria. Exclusion criteria are characteristics that you purposely do not wish to include in your search; for example, white people with diabetes if the problem pertains to Afro-Caribbean males with diabetes. Both inclusion and exclusion criteria are important characteristics of a research study; they have implications for both the interpretation and the generalisability of the findings (Polit and Beck, 2011).

 When I was on a theory block at the university, the library ran a workshop on accessing the databases specifically for nursing students. I went on the session, it was about 3 hours all in all and it was just so helpful, I would recommend this to anyone. If they run one next semester I will also go on that as a refresher.
Aaron, first year student nurse

SECTION SUMMARY

There are many sources the nurse can draw upon to access the evidence to support a care intervention or care regimen and sometimes this can seem quite daunting. Devising and honing an answerable question from the outset helps to reduce the amount of core evidence. You should be prepared to go back to the question, reconsider the choice of keywords and refine them, becoming more specific as you do so. The judicious use of inclusion and exclusion criteria will help you focus. Remember to record all of your searches as you work through the task.

Barriers to implementing evidence-based practice

EBP is not the key to all the problems that you will face in your attempts to provide high-quality, safe and cost-effective care. Just as there are barriers that prevent nurses from using research in everyday practice, this is also true of implementing EBP. The following factors may hinder and have a negative impact:

- lack of value for or disregard of research in clinical practice,
- challenges in changing practice,
- availability of knowledgeable mentors,
- time to conduct research,
- lack of education concerning the research process,
- lack of understanding and awareness about research or EBP,
- research reports/articles not readily accessible,
- challenges in accessing research reports and articles,
- no time to read research,
- complexity of research reports,
- lack of knowledge about EBP and ability to critique articles,
- feeling overwhelmed by the process.

Regardless of these barriers and the challenges they bring, nurses are participating in EBP and having a positive impact in patient outcomes. Barriers can be overcome when organisational efforts focus on integrating research in practice and use strategies such as journal clubs, nursing grand rounds and having research articles available for review (Fink *et al.*, 2005).

PEARLS OF WISDOM

To be successful with EBP you must be ready to challenge your own assumptions and willing to work with others to improve care processes and patient outcomes.

EBP requires resources, work, time and effort, but the outcomes make them worthwhile. Each patient deserves care that is grounded on the best scientific knowledge available, ensuring high-quality, safe and cost-effective care.

 ## Summary

Nurses should draw on all of the various sources of evidence available and understand how to find and access the evidence, what to do with it once it has been located and how to apply it to their practice. These are the hallmarks of a professional, enabling the nurse to assure patients that the care provided is safe and effective. All healthcare professionals including nurses need to engage with EBP owing to the increasing complexity of healthcare and the need to comply with codes of conduct. They must make informed judgements about the care provided. EBP does not mean that evidence is used only to change practice; it is also there to support existing practice.

 ## References

Berwick, D. M. (2003) Disseminating innovations in health care. *Journal of the American Medical Association* 289(15), 1969–75

Burns, N. and Grove, S.K. (2011) *Understanding Nursing Research*, 4th edn. Elsevier. Philadelphia

Canadian Medical Association Journal (1979) The Periodic Health Examination. Canadian Task Force on the Periodic Health Examination. *Canadian Medical Association Journal* 121(9), 1193–1254

Carnwell, R. (2001) Essential differences between research and evidence-based practice. *Nurse Researcher* 8(2), 55–68

Carper, B. (1978) Fundamental patterns of knowing in nursing. *Advances in Nursing Science* 1(1), 13–23

Greenberg, M. and Pyle, B. (2004) Achieving evidence-based nursing practice in ambulatory care. *Viewpoint* 26(1), 8–12

Fink, R., Thompson, C.J. and Bonnes, D. (2005) Overcoming barriers and promoting the use of research in practice. *Journal of Nursing Administration* 35(3), 121–9

Griffiths, P. (2006) What does evidence-based practice mean? *Journal of Advanced Perioperative Care* 2(4), 137–41

Hurley, W.L., Denegar, C.R. and Hertel, J. (2011) *Research Methods. A Framework for Evidence-Based Clinical Practice*. Lippincott, Philadelphia

Jolley, J. (2010) *Introducing Research and Evidence-Based Practice for Nurses*. Pearson, Harlow

Larrabee, J.H. (2009) *Nurse to Nurse. Evidence Based Practice*. McGraw Hill, New York

Mantzoukas, S. (2007) A review of evidence-based practice, nursing research and reflection: leveling the hierarchy. *Journal of Clinical Nursing* 17(2), 214–23

Muir Gray, J.A. (1997) *Evidence Based Healthcare: How to Make Health Policy and Management Decision*. Churchill Livingstone, Edinburgh

Newell, R. and Burnard, P. (2011) *Research for Evidence-Based Practice in Healthcare*, 2nd edn. Wiley Blackwell, Oxford

Nursing and Midwifery Council (2008) *The Code: Standards of Conduct, Performance and Ethics for Nurses and Midwives.* Nursing and Midwifery Council, London

Nursing and Midwifery Council (2010) *Pre Registration Nursing Education in the UK.* http://standards.nmc-uk.org/Documents/Pre-registration%20nursing%20education%20in%20UK%20FINAL%2006092010.pdf

O'Halloran, P. (2010) Evidence based practice and its critics: what is a nurse manager to do? *Journal of Nursing Management* 18(1), 90–5

Petticrew, M. and Roberts, H. (2003) Evidence, hierarchies and typologies: horses for courses. *Journal of Epidemiology and Community Health* 57, 527–9

Polit, D.F. and Beck, C.T. (2011) *Nursing Research: Generating and Accessing Evidence for Nursing Practice*, 9th edn. Lippincott, Philadelphia

Rycroft-Malone, J., Harvey, J.G. and Seers, K. (2004) An explanation of the factors that influence the implementation of evidence into practice. *Journal of Clinical Nursing* 13(8), 913–24

Sears, S. (2006) The role of information technology in evidence-based practice. *Clinical Nurse Specialist* 20(1), 7–8

Sackett, D.L. (1994) Cochrane Collaboration. *British Medical Journal* 306(6967), 1514–15

Sackett, D.L., Rosenberg, W.M., Gray, J.A. and Haynes, R.B. (1996) Evidence based medicine: what it is and what it isn't. *British Medical Journal* 312(7023), 71–2

Straus, S.E., Glasziou, P., Richardson, W.S. and Haynes, R.B. (2011) *Evidence-Based Medicine. How to Practice and Teach It*, 4th edn. Elsevier, Edinburgh

 ## Resources

Centre for Evidence-based Medicine

www.cebm.net/index.aspx?o=1157

The Centre for Evidence-based Medicine provides free support and resources to doctors, clinicians, teachers and others interested in learning more about evidence-based medicine.

Clinical Evidence

www.clinicalevidence.com/x/index.html

Clinical Evidence comprises a database of high-quality, rigorously developed systematic overviews assessing the benefits and harms of treatments and a suite of evidence-based medicine resources and training materials. You have to register to access this resource

Guideline and Audit Implementation Network

www.gain-ni.org/

GAIN's main function is to promote leadership in safety and quality of care through the development and integration of regional guidelines and audit and their implementation to improve outcomes for patients, clients and carers.

National Institute for Health and Clinical Excellence

www.nice.org.uk

See Resources section in Chapter 5

NHS Evidence

www.library.nhs.uk

NHS Evidence is a service that enables access to authoritative clinical and non-clinical evidence and best practice through a web-based portal. It helps people from across the NHS, public health and social care sectors to make better clinical decisions.

PRODIGY

http://prodigy.clarity.co.uk/home

PRODIGY is a service that aims to provide a reliable source of evidence-based information and guidance about the common conditions managed in primary and first-contact care. It helps healthcare professionals and patients make evidence-based decisions about healthcare and provides them with the know-how to put these decisions into practice.

Scottish Intercollegiate Guidelines Network

www.sign.ac.uk

See Resources section in Chapter 5

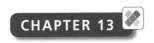

CHAPTER 13

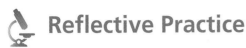

Reflective Practice

> **WHAT THIS CHAPTER CONTAINS**
>
> - Defining key terms
> - What reflection is and what it is not
> - Models of reflection
> - The value of reflection
> - Practical issues

This chapter provides you with essential information concerning reflective practice. It takes years to refine and hone the skills required to be a good reflective practitioner.

Defining reflection

Reflection means different things to different people, but in a nutshell it is about working through, thinking purposefully about and critically analysing actions you have taken with the aim of changing and improving your practice. Far more articulate definitions are available and include one from Boud *et al.* (1985), who stated that:

> Reflection is a forum of response of the learner to experience.

This is about involving yourself in the learning process. Learning comes from within and comprises the self and is generated by asking questions concering actions, values and beliefs, and sometimes this is difficult. There are a number of essential stages or elements associated with the act of effective reflection. For example:

- being mindful of any uncomfortable feelings and thoughts,
- using critical analysis and attending to your feelings,
- growing, doing more learning associated with a new perspective on the situation.

Reflection is multifaceted; it is not just about looking in a mirror! It is a complex concept and therefore coming to one fixed definition is impossible, but among all

---

The Student Nurse Toolkit: An Essential Guide for Surviving Your Course, First Edition. Ian Peate.

of the definitions that do exist there are some commonalities. An understanding of the purpose of reflective practice and its components can be acquired by considering some of the definitions provided in the literature. These are some definitions you might find useful.

- 'Reflection is a process of reviewing an experience of practice in order to describe, analyse, evaluate and so inform learning about practice' (Reid, 1993).
- 'Reflective practice is something more than thoughtful practice. It is that form of practice that seeks to problematise many situations of professional performance so that they can become potential learning situations and so the practitioner can continue to learn, grow and develop in and through practice' (Jarvis, 1992).
- 'A window through which the practitioner can view and focus self within the context of his/her own lived experience in ways that enable him/her to confront, understand and work towards resolving the contradictions within his/her practice between what is desirable and actual practice' (Johns 2000).

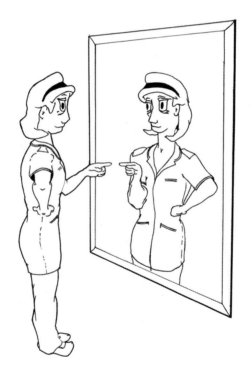

Such an array of definitions to choose from can help or hinder you in your quest to get to grips with this important activity. Choose a definition that closely aligns to the one that is preferred in your university, but be aware that there are other definitions available.

Duffy (2007) notes that reflective practice is an active, thoughtful process of examining practice in a critical way. The individual is challenged and empowered to undertake the process of self-enquiry to allow the person to realise desirable and effective practice within a reflexive spiral of personal change. Bolton (2010) adds that reflection is a state of mind where the person reflecting pays particular attention to the practical values and theories that inform everyday actions, leading to developmental insight.

> **If I am asked to reflect any more I will turn into a mirror.**
> *Kofi, first year student nurse*

SECTION SUMMARY

There are a number of definitions of reflection. Reflection provides the nurse with an opportunity to consciously think about what they have done and what they might do. Reflective practice is only as good as the person doing the reflection.

 ## Reflection: what it is and what it is not

Nurses (those who are registered and those undertaking a programme of study to become registered) are required to draw on a number of personal qualities on a daily basis. Box 13.1 provides you with a list of some of them.

Box 13.1 Personal qualities

A concern for individuals: does the care of those people around you matter to you? Are you concerned about what happens to them?

A curiosity about people: are you curious about how other people think and feel? Do you take an interest in what they say and do?

An enquiring mind: are you enquiring? Do you have a desire to find out more about things that interest you? Are you keen to dig deeper, to analyse and to build on the knowledge you already have?

A logical approach: do you want to establish facts, test out ideas, discover how things work and determine why things go wrong, why they went wrong? Do you approach problems in a logical and sensible manner?

An open mind: do you respect people whose values and beliefs, attitudes and background are very different from yours? Do you have the ability to see things from other perspectives, from other people's point of view?

Creativity and imagination: do you see problems and actively seek to find new solutions? Do you think of responses to challenging issues that other people may not have thought of?

Able to manage pressure: how have you had to cope with highly pressured situations? Did this affect the way you behaved or did you manage to handle it?

Hard work: are you able to cope with hard work over continual periods of time? Do you have stamina?

Tolerance: do you become impatient with others easily, or can you go along at their pace while still being considerate?

Grit: if something does not come right first time, do you give up or devote time and effort to sorting it out so it does come right?

Decisiveness: do you make decisions with confidence, based on what you know and seeking more information if needed?

Modesty: are you able and content to recognise your own limits? Can you, and do you, look to others for help?

Reflecting appropriately will help you understand where your strengths are and where you are not so strong, and help you work more effectively in a multidisciplinary team.

ACTIVITY 13.1

Of the qualities listed in Box 13.1 which ones do you recognise in yourself? What do you do well? What could be improved upon? Do any of them not apply to you and, if so, why not?

Reflective practice can help you delve deeper. It can help you become more curious about yourself but it cannot change you. You are the only person who can do that (if change is needed). Reflection encourages us to become aware of our thoughts (intellectual) and feelings (affective) related to a particular learning experience or area of practice.

Learning emerges as a result of our experiences; however, it does not just materialise. For effective learning to take place you have to engage in reflection and to record your reflections. Experiences are translated into meaningful learning when you think about what you are doing as well as why you are doing it. As a professional and a reflective practitioner you can use that learning to increase your professional knowledge and skills. In turn this helps you develop personally and will also be of benefit to the people and families for whom you care.

Looking back on a situation begins the process of reflection; this entails taking deliberate time to think it over, learning from it and then using that learning to help you in future, should similar situations arise. Reflection, which is learning through experience, is not a new concept. We reflect on our surroundings and experiences on a daily basis. Moon (2004, 2007) suggest that it is the conscious, deliberate and ordered process of using reflection as a learning tool in our professional practice that is more of a challenge. It is a complex activity requiring the individual to create a set of skills needed for problem solving.

Reflective practice is not the panacea for the ills that befall nurses or nursing. It can only help you become more critical, analysing your own experience with the aim of generating evidence from your own practice (Jasper and Rolfe, 2011). Reflective practice is about learning from experience. It generates locally owned knowledge, but it does not separate practice and theory (Ghaye and Lillyman, 2010).

Benner *et al.* (1996) point out that something that seems straightforward in the science laboratory or textbook may not be so clear when you are at the bedside. Reflective practice in this sense can be seen as a bridge between theory and practice: it has the potential to be a powerful means of using theory to inform practice.

PEARLS OF WISDOM

When you begin the reflective process be sure to:
- be spontaneous, impulsive,
- articulate yourself freely,
- have an open mind,
- choose the time to reflect that suits you,
- prepare yourself personally,
- (if appropriate) choose your own reflective model, one that resonates with you.

Reflective models

The previous section of this chapter demonstrated that learning comes about when you reflect, or more correctly it has the potential to come about if the reflective process is carried out in a coherent, structured way. The use of models can help your reflection become more structured rather than being ad hoc.

Models are only theoretical principles that come together as one practical whole. They are idealisations that have the ability to help you understand, but they do not describe and most importantly they do not tell you how you act.

ACTIVITY 13.2

If you are familiar with the London underground you may have used a two-dimensional model: the route map of the various lines.

Have a look at the London underground map and plan your route from Kings Cross to Paddington. Having done that, get hold of copy of a London street map and plan the same route. You will see that the underground map is a topological map rather than a true representation of the underground system. It merely serves to help you get from station A to station B.

 Models and frameworks

There are different types of reflection and the distinction between them needs to be made. Reflection can be described in two key ways:

- ☒ reflection *in* action,
- ☒ reflection *on* action.

Looking back after the event is reflection *on* action, and reflection *in* action happens during the event. There are a number of different interpretations of reflection on action.

> I am in my third year and it is only now that I fully appreciate how helpful reflection is. Previously it was a chore but now I am much more comfortable with it. The effort is worth it.
> *Sue, third year student*

Greenwood (1993) suggests that reflection *in* action means thinking about what you are doing when you are doing it and it often comes about by surprise. It gives you the opportunity to reshape what you are doing while you are doing it (Benner *et al.*, 1996). This is about thinking on your feet.

Reflection *on* action occurs when you look back, contemplating your practice with the intention of uncovering the knowledge used in practical situations. It happens when you analyse and interpret the information (Fitzgerald, 1994). In reflection *on* action the information gained is turned into knowledge and permits us to challenge concepts and theories, looking at things in different ways.

When you reflect in writing this is usually about you reflecting *on* action. To reflect *on* and *in* action you need to make plans about your reflection prior to acting.

 ## Kolb's learning cycle

There are times when you will reflect alone; however, reflection also involves a dialogue between yourself and your peers, lecturers, practice learning facilitators, work-placement tutors and, in some instances, patients and their families. All of these can provide you with useful feedback required for reflection. Kolb (1984) has developed a learning cycle; this is a simple and useful tool illuminating the connection between reflection and improved learning (see Figure 13.1).

Kolb's learning cycle is based on the principle that reflective practice does not occur as a one-off event. Rather, it is an ongoing cyclical process of experiencing, observing, theorising and making active plans. Reflection occurs as you are moving through each part of the process. The way this model is used depends on individual experience and interpretation as well as the amount of time it takes to complete the cycle.

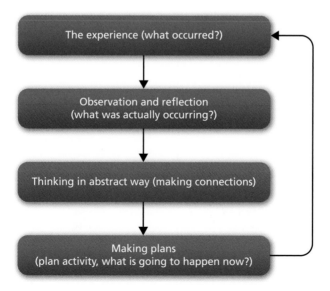

Figure 13.1 A learning cycle. *Source*: data from Kolb (1984).

Gibbs' reflective cycle

Gibbs (1988) proposed a reflective cycle that begins with describing an event and then works through the following stages in turn. This model is a popular model that is used for reflection; it has a six-step process and is one of the few models that encourages you to take your emotions into account (see Figure 13.2).

Each of the stages in this model asks you a question, as follows.

Describe: what happened? At this point do not make any judgements, do not try and come to any conclusions: just describe.

Feel: what were your thoughts and feelings at the time? Do not try or begin to analyse yet, just capture your thoughts and feelings.

Evaluate: take some time now to think about what was good or bad about the experience. Evaluate the way the experience made you feel and react, so that now you can make value judgements.

Analyse: what sense (if any) can you make of the situation? You can bring in ideas from outside of the experience to help here. Consider what was really going on (remember this is about the whole experience). Did any other people (maybe your peers) experience similar or different things to you? Did they differ or were they similar? If the former, how did they differ? In your analysis, were there any themes that began to emerge?

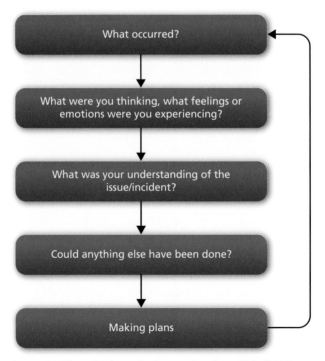

Figure 13.2 The reflective cycle. *Source*: data from Gibbs (1998).

Deduce: having analysed so far, was there anything that could be deduced (generally) from the experience? Now move on to the more specific: this is now about you. What can be determined by your own specific, unique, personal situation or your way of working?

Action plan: the final stage is the development of personal action plans. Now ask yourself what you might do differently in this situation next time. What steps might you take based on your learning?

ACTIVITY 13.3

Think about a recent *non-clincal* experience that you have had and apply Gibbs' reflective cycle to it.

Phase	Prompt	Your notes
Description	What happened? Describe the situation. Do not form any opinions yet or come to any conclusions.	
Feelings	What where your thoughts and feelings at the time? (Just note them at this point.)	
Evaluation	What were the good and bad things about this experience? Begin now to make value judgements. Evaluate the way the experience made you feel and react.	
Analysis	What sense can you make of the experience? What do you think was really going on? Do others feel the same as you?	
Deductions	What conclusions can you make about the whole situation, generally? Was there anything in the experience about you and your own specific, unique, personal situation or your way of working?	
Action planning	Given the total experience and all the learning that has happened, what might you do differently next time (if anything)?	

> We use Gibbs' cycle at our university, I like it, it makes me think things through logically. *Gillie, third year student nurse*

The five Rs of reflection

Earlier in this chapter it was emphasised that a systemic approach to reflection is considered useful as it helps you to work through the situation or the experience. Using a framework can help. One that encourages deep and purposeful thinking about what happened is the five Rs of reflection framework (see Figure 13.3), from the work of Bain *et al.* (2002). The five Rs are:

- 🎗 reporting,
- 🎗 responding,
- 🎗 relating,
- 🎗 reasoning,
- 🎗 reconstructing.

Table 13.1 considers some triggers that may help you when thinking about using the five Rs of reflection.

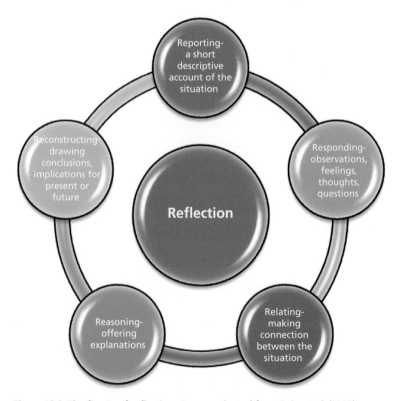

Figure 13.3 The five Rs of reflection. *Source*: adapted from Bain *et al.* (2002).

Table 13.1 Triggers associated with the five Rs

The five Rs	Trigger
Reporting	What happened and what did the issue involve? What was I doing at the time? Where was I? When did the issue occur? Was anyone else involved, if so who? How was I involved in the issue? What was significant? What do I need to pay attention to?
Responding	Did it go well or not? How was my performance? How do I know if it worked (or didn't)? Specifically, what worked well? How do I know that it worked well? Specifically, what worked least well? What makes me think that? How was I feeling, and was there anything that made me feel that way? How do I think others were feeling and what might have made them feel that way? How was my emotional response, how was my personal response and what did my behaviours tell of how I responded to the issues?
Relating	What theoretical perspective or body of knowledge are relevant to the issue and why? How does the theory relate to my personal and professional experiences and in what way?
Reasoning	Do I have an explanation or reason for what occurred? How do the theory and the research enlighten my thinking about this issue? What is the impact of different perspectives; for example, on and by my peers?
Reconstructing	All in all, what are my thoughts about this issue? Are there any conclusions that I can make from the issue? How can I justify them? Looking back, is there anything I would do differently next time, and why? Has this issue taught me anything about myself? Has this issue taught me anything about my professional practice? In what ways can I use this experience to enhance care provision in the future?

Source: adapted Bain *et al.* (2002).

ACTIVITY 13.4

Think about an incident where you might apply the five Rs.
Use the prompts for the five Rs in Table 13.1. Was this helpful?
Did it help you organise your thoughts and feelings?

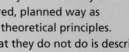

SECTION SUMMARY

Models and frameworks will only provide you with a way of reflecting on your practice in a structured, planned way as opposed to an ad hoc way. Models are theoretical principles. They can help you understand, but what they do not do is describe or tell you how you should behave. The five Rs of reflection can help you work through a situation or experience systematically.

The value of reflection

In a profession as challenging as nursing, honest self-reflection is central. This means that we must regularly examine what has worked and what has not. It can sometimes be painful to look into a mirror and see what is facing you. Undergraduate nursing programmes require that you are able to demonstrate competence in the ability to reflect effectively on your practice (Nursing and Midwifery Council, 2010).

PEARLS OF WISDOM

Reflective practice you can:
- enhance patient care,
- bring new insight and new ideas,
- acquire new understanding,
- take a step back and think about a situation,
- gain new perspectives,
- make sense of your experiences and construct meaning and knowledge that helps guide actions.

Practical issues

As you go through your undergraduate programme of study you will be introduced constantly to a mass of theoretical knowledge and new practice experiences. One way of helping you link the theory to practice is through reflection helping to integrate learning. You will accomplish a great deal of this learning by being actively involved in the practice of reflection. From a practical perspective you can:

- become more self-aware (see Chapter 10),
- direct your thoughts and feelings on your experiences,
- develop a wider, greater, understanding of health and social care practices,
- appreciate and recognise the knowledge and skills that you have and what you have developed,

- recognise what your strengths are and any areas that may require growth,
- create an action plan for future practice, updating and amending it as required.

Your programme of study may determine what you are required to reflect on and you should find out about this. In general, you can reflect on any theoretical or practice experience associated with your professional and personal development. Reflections can be associated with positive or negative experiences and can include:

- an activity or interaction that left you feeling happy or unhappy,
- an incident that raised a moral or ethical dilemma,
- examples of your practice,
- events that are memorable,
- the learning of a new skill,
- the development of learned skills,
- an event that caused frustration,
- any occurrence where you developed your knowledge, skills and attitudes,
- any event where you were able to make the link between practice and theory.

Reflective writing

You are required to develop and provide evidence on your programme of study that your writing skills have advanced. This includes the skills of reflective writing. As you develop these skills will also develop and grow and you will become more familiar with them as you progress as a student and as a practitioner.

Jasper (2011) notes that reflective writing is a skill that can be learned and improved with practice. Reflective writing may be a core feature in most or all of your assignments and you must follow any guidelines offered on your course. Your reflective writing is evidence of your reflective thinking. Reflective thinking usually involves:

- looking back at something, usually an event; for example, something that happened;
- thinking in depth and from different perspectives about the event, endeavouring to explain it, usually with reference to a theoretical model;
- taking time to think carefully about what the event or idea meant for you and your ongoing progress.

These are some practical suggestions that may help you when writing in an academic context. This type of writing is more personal than the other kinds of academic writing that you may be asked to produce. When you think in a reflective way, particularly if done in discussion with others, it is often unstructured and the dialogue flows freely. When you write reflectively – for example, as part of an assignment – it is usual for it to be done in a structured way.

There are a number of ways of structuring reflective writing and you may be required to follow a particular model. Try to remember the following points when submitting assessed work that is based on reflection:

- ☒ you are required to do more than describe events: reflection requires you to explore and provide an explanation of events;
- ☒ it is expected that you will disclose anxieties, concerns, mistakes and weaknesses;
- ☒ it is envisaged that you should be able to demonstrate some understanding of likely causes and to explain how you plan to improve;
- ☒ usually you are expected to select just the most meaningful parts of the event on which you are reflecting. Attempting to discuss the whole event may mean that you will not have enough space to do it justice and the outcome will be a superficial discussion.

 ## Gather your ideas

Prior to putting pen to paper, you need to think and reflect. You can start this process by drawing a mindmap. This is a technique that can help you develop your thinking, organise your ideas and make connections.

- ☒ Write the issue in the centre of a blank page.
- ☒ Draw related ideas on 'branches' radiating from the central topic. When a new idea comes to you, start a new branch from the centre. You should include any ideas, topics, authors and theories, and experiences associated with your issue.
- ☒ Do the mapping quickly, trying not to pause. This will help you maintain a flow of ideas. Just put any ideas down at this point: anything and everything is acceptable, and try to not self-edit.
- ☒ Circle the key points or ideas. Look at each item and think about how it relates to others and to the issue as a whole.
- ☒ Map the relationships between the ideas or key points, using lines, arrows and colours. Use words or phrases to link them.

 I hate using mindmaps they don't help me at all.
James, second year student nurse

 We used mindmaps in sixth form, I find them really useful. They help me plan, focus and structure; they are not for everyone.
Tammy, first year student nurse

Reflective writing assignments can take a number of forms (see Table 13.2), and you are advised to check the guidelines provided in your programme outline prior to beginning. If you have any queries or concerns then be sure to clarify them with your lecturer or personal tutor. There may be a course requirement that stipulates how you are required to submit your work; for example, as a book or folder or by completing an online component. Clarify whether you are permitted to include pictures, diagrams or media clippings to supplement and support you submission.

Table 13.2 Types of reflective writing assignment

Type	Description
Journal	You may be expected to write weekly entries throughout the term. Your reflections may need to be based on course content.
Learning diary	This is similar to a journal, but may entail group participation. The diary then becomes the place for you to communicate with other members of the group.
Log book	You note down or record (log) what you have done. This provides you with an accurate record of a process, helping you reflect on past actions and make better decisions for future actions.
Reflective note	A reflective note that encourages you to think about your personal reaction to a professional issue raised in your course.
Essay diary	This approach may take the form of an annotated bibliography (sources of evidence you might include in your essay) and a critique (reflecting on your own writing and research processes).
Peer review	Involves students showing their work to their peers for feedback.
Self-assessment	You are required to comment on your own work.

You must ensure that you adhere to the guidelines concerning confidentiality in your course handbook. Failure to comply with confidentiality guidelines could result in automatic failure.

Reflective writing is not about conveying information, instruction or argument. Although there may be descriptive elements in your writing, this is not about pure description. Reflection is not a summary of course notes or a standard university essay, it is more about your responses to experiences, and your thoughts and feelings. It will become a way of thinking to explore your learning, an approach to help you make meaning out of what it is you study.

SECTION SUMMARY

There are a variety of practical issues that need to be taken into account to ensure that all of your efforts come to fruition, enabling you to link theory to practice. Reflective writing is a skill that can be learned and improved with practice. Prior to writing a reflective account you need to think and reflect; there are a number of techniques that can help your thinking. Reflective writing assignments take a number of forms; check the guidelines provided by your university before you begin writing.

Summary

Reflection is not a new concept, but it can take time to master. It is a process that is undertaken in a conscious manner to gain further understanding and add meaning to our lives. Reflection is very closely aligned with learning through experience and has the potential to help us make sense of and learn from situations in which we have been involved: good and bad, comfortable and uncomfortable.

When we reflect it helps us to think, and to explore our thoughts and feelings, working through an experience, with the aim of gaining new understandings, new insights and deeper self-awareness. Reflection is not a passive activity but comprises actively considering and learning from our thoughts and deeds, and using them as a vehicle for advancing reflective thinking.

Engaging in reflective practice can assist you with your ongoing personal and professional learning; through it you can demonstrate your ability to achieve the learning outcomes and standards of competence as demanded by the NMC. As a registered practitioner you are required to demonstrate on going competence (see Chapter 18). Evidence of meaningful and insightful reflective practice can provide that necessary proof.

References

Bain, J.D., Ballantyne, R., Mills, C. and Lester, N.C. (2002) *Reflecting on Practice: Student Teachers' Perspectives*. Post Pressed, Flaxton

Benner, P., Tanner, C.A. and Chesla, C.A. (1996) *Expertise in Nursing: Caring, Clinical Judgement and Ethics*. Springer, New York

Bolton, G. (2010) *Reflective Practice. Writing and Professional Development*, 3rd edn. Sage, London

Boud, D., Keogh, R. and Walker, D. (1985) *Reflection: Turning Experience into Learning*. Kogan Page, London

Duffy, A. (2007). A *Concept Analysis of Reflective Practice: Determining its Value to Nurses*. *British Journal of Nursing* 16(22), 1400–7

Fitzgerald, M. (1994) Theories of reflection for learning. In Palmer, A. and Burns, S. (eds), *Reflective Practice in Nursing*. Blackwell Scientific, Oxford, pp. 63–84

Gibbs, G. (1998) *Learning by Doing: A Guide to Teaching and Learning Methods*. Further Education Unit Oxford Polytechnic, Oxford

Ghaye, T. and Lillyman, S. (2010) *Reflection: Principles and Practices for Healthcare Professionals*. Quay Books, London

Greenwood, J. (1993) Reflective practice a critique of the work of Argyris and Schon. *Journal of Advanced Nursing* 18(8), 1183–7

Jasper, M. (2011) Understanding reflective writing. In Rolfe, G., Jasper, M. and Freshwater, D. (eds), *Critical Reflection in Practice. Generating Knowledge for Care*, 2nd edn. Palgrave, Basingstoke, pp. 52–73

Jasper, M. and Rolfe, G. (2011) Critical reflection and the emergence of professional knowledge. In Rolfe, G., Jasper, M. and Freshwater, D. (eds), *Critical Reflection in Practice. Generating Knowledge for Care*, 2nd edn. Palgrave, Basingstoke, pp. 1–10

Kolb, D.A. (1984) *Experiential Learning: Experience as the Source of Learning and Development.* Prentice-Hall, New Jersey

Moon, J.A. (2004). *A Handbook of Reflective and Experiential Learning: Theory and Practice.* Routledge, London

Moon, J.A. (2007) *Reflection and Employability.* Learning Teaching and Support Network, York

Nursing and Midwifery Council (2010) *Standards for Pre Registration Nursing Education.* http://standards.nmc-uk.org/PublishedDocuments/Standards%20for%20pre-registration%20nursing%20education%2016082010.pdf

Reid, B. (1993) 'But we're doing it already!' Exploring a response to the concept of reflective practice in order to improve its facilitation. *Nurse Education Today* 13, 305–9

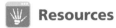 ## Resources

Health Education Academy

www.heacademy.ac.uk

Provides resources to support the higher education community to enhance the quality and impact of learning and teaching.

Skills Academy

www.skillsacademyforhealth.org.uk

Created to help the healthcare sector develop a range of skills, with the ultimate aim of making employees more valuable to employers.

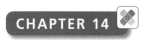

CHAPTER 14

Your Professional Portfolio

- Description of a professional portfolio
- The need for a professional portfolio
- The structure and content of a professional portfolio
- Professional portfolio formats

Some undergraduate nursing programmes require students to develop and main-tain a professional portfolio. They can also be called personal development port-folios or simply portfolios and there are many ways in which they can be achieved. The professional portfolio can take the form of a reflective document that is linked with the achievements of the NMC competencies (Nursing and Midwifery Council, 2010). In some universities completion of the portfolio is a compulsory aspect of the programme and a prerequisite for each progression point: it is seen as a tool for knowledge management, providing a link between the individual and organ-isational learning.

The use of professional portfolios in documenting competence is becoming increasingly common in pre-registration graduate nursing programmes and is also being used more and more by some employers. The professional portfolio is rec-ognised as an important means of documenting and evaluating achievements and improvements in student learning. The use of technology has enabled a wider range of people to assess student achievement; for example, professional bodies and future employers.

Confidentiality

You are required to ensure that no part of any of your records (in whatever for-mat) discloses the name or makes identifiable any person you have cared for, their families or colleagues. Because of this you must take care when writing any records or making public any information associated with your professional portfolio (or other records). This applies to verbal communcation too, such as when discussing any issues relating to any record with mentors or personal tutors that in any way relates to service users, clients or colleagues.

The professional portfolio

A portfolio is something that demonstrates learning from experience. It enables an assessor to measure learning, acts as a vehicle for reflective thinking, highlights critical analysis skills and provides evidence of self-directed learning accompanied by a collection of evidence surrounding a person's competence (Scholes *et al.*, 2004). Timmins and Duffy (2011) describe a portfolio, based on the Latin translation of the word, to mean, in general, a receptacle for information. Farrell (2008) notes that the literature is replete with definitions and descriptions of portfolios and that as such there is often ambiguity concerning the different terms. The professional portfolio is more than just a portfolio or a record of continuing professional development (or CPD) that includes certificates, diplomas and other documents. It is an organised collection of evidence that sums up what you have learned from your prior experience through reflection and what it is you intend to learn and excel in: your aim, objectives and aspirations.

> I feel that my whole life is in my professional portfolio; I go over it regularly, adding and adding to it. I feel really proud of what I have achieved and I know there is more to achieve. My portfolio is my story about me. *Jorge, third year student nurse*

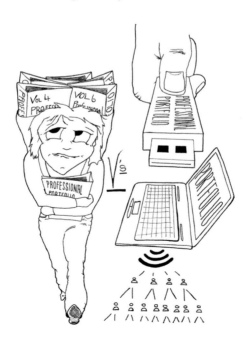

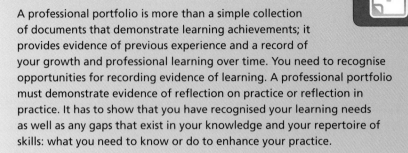

SECTION SUMMARY

A professional portfolio is more than a simple collection of documents that demonstrate learning achievements; it provides evidence of previous experience and a record of your growth and professional learning over time. You need to recognise opportunities for recording evidence of learning. A professional portfolio must demonstrate evidence of reflection on practice or reflection in practice. It has to show that you have recognised your learning needs as well as any gaps that exist in your knowledge and your repertoire of skills: what you need to know or do to enhance your practice.

The need for a professional portfolio

The rationale for completing and maintaining a professional portfolio is varied. It can help you demonstrate, through the gathering of appropriate evidence, how the competencies and the essential skills clusters inherent in your progamme of study have been achieved over the 3 years (Nursing and Midwifery Council, 2010). The professional portfolio should be seen as a critical component of your nurse education programme.

PEARLS OF WISDOM

The professional portfolio is basically what an abstract is to a journal article. It provides your lecturer and your future employer with a description of who you are and how you reached registration.

Like other professionals, nurses need to provide evidence of their growth and achievement over time: the public expects this. The professional portfolio is a vehicle for collecting and presenting that evidence. Currently, registered nurses are required by the NMC to undertake and record their CPD over the 3 years prior to the renewal of their registration (Nursing and Midwifery Council, 2011). This may be done through the maintenance of a professional portfolio of learning activities that are relevant to their sphere of practice.

Clark (2010a) notes that professional portfolios for registered nurses and student nurses are key resources required to record developing skills and knowledge, as well as details about career progression. The success of the portfolio will be associated with what constitutes meaningful evidence of achievement and how to structure the portfolio to best represent development: personally and professionally.

PEARLS OF WISDOM

When nurses examine their own practices carefully, those practices are likely to improve.

The professional portfolio provides evidence of your previous experiences and presents a dynamic and fluid record of your growth and professional learning. Coffey (2005) refers to this as a series of snapshots over time, representative of the person's experiences and learning from and about practice. It has already been said that there are many reasons why a professional portfolio is constructed and maintained. One of its prime purposes is to allow you to show or display achievements of professional competence, learning outcomes and knowledge development. It is your showcase. This interpretation of a professional portfolio is more comprehensive than the portfolio definition (a collection of papers). The professional portfolio relates to your professional role as a nurse.

When you think about your practice (reflecting) and you develop a portfolio as a result of this thinking your learning becomes more explicit as you translate your clinical experiences into evidence that is documented (Timmins and Duffy, 2011). Critically examining your learning related to the specific experiences as you practice demonstrates the learning that has taken place as a result of those experiences.

Twadell and Johnson (2007) suggest that portfolios help you demonstrate your reflective skills, critical thinking skills, decision-making skills, problem-solving skills and interpersonal skills, as well as indicating the range of clinical skills you have mastered and are developing. The portfolio allows you to demonstrate your progression from novice to expert nurse throughout your nursing career (see Figure 14.1) (see also Chapter 10).

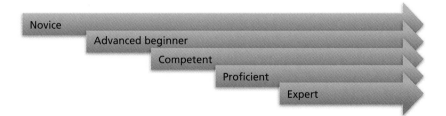

Figure 14.1 Levels of competence. *Source*: data from Benner (1984).

> We started putting together our professional portfolio from day one of the course. It was a good idea to introduce it so early. I took my portfolio to a job interview last week and the panel was really impressed with the contents, so I am happy the university kept banging on about it. I got the job, by the way.
>
> *Jay, third year student*

There is a range of reasons why nursing students (and healthcare practitioners) are required to put together a professional portfolio and this includes the need to:

- gain and maintain a license or registration to practice, as required by the regulator (the NMC),
- renew nursing registration: this requires a statement or portfolio about your competence to practice; you may be audited to provide evidence of this,
- provide evidence of focusing on professional educational needs,
- demonstrate levels of performance against organisational requirements,
- demonstrate that you are up to date with developments in your field of practice.

A professional portfolio will help you to demonstrate that you understand the following.

- As a registered nurse you will have significant responsibilities in the provision of healthcare interventions with the aim of protecting patients from the effects of illness and disability and promoting health and well-being. It is unacceptable to do things 'the way they always have been done' or 'because that's how we do things here'.
- You keep yourself informed about knowledge development and recommended practice changes relevant to your current and future role as the provision of healthcare becomes increasingly complex due to changes in epidemiology, technology, pharmacology, health systems and the role of the nurse.
- You possess the knowledge and skills to provide safe and effective care.
- You recognise and value the concept of lifelong learning. Professional portfolios are a way of demonstrating continuous learning, that you are a lifelong learner.
- You reflect on your practice to continually improve your practice.

 Personal development planning

Personal development planning (PDP) is a method or framework to help you identify your strengths and to determine areas in your learning that need further development. Reed (2011) suggests that for the professional portfolio to demonstrate your learning successfully you must capture both the planned and the unexpected.

The Quality Assurance Agency for Higher Education (2009) defines the PDP as a structured process that is undertaken by the learner with support to enable them to reflect on their own learning, their performance and their ability to plan for the future; that is, their personal, educational and career development. Each educational institution is required to provide structured and supported opportunities for PDP. PDP is often used in combination with a professional portfolio, providing you with skills and a foundation for similar processes required by future employers. This can help you achieve your full potential personally, professionally and academically but, to get the most out of it, you have to be committed.

The steps of the PDP cycle

There are a number of steps associated with the PDP cycle that can help you in managing your personal, professional and academic development. Each university adopts its own approach, but there are similarities across institutions. Five key steps make up the cycle, occurring in a specific sequence. Regardless of the step, previous steps can be re-visited and the concluding step leads back to the first step but at a higher level (see Table 14.1).

Table 14.1 Five steps associated with the PDP cycle

Step	Description
Self-assessment	Compilation of information allowing you to judge where it is you are now from a personal, academic and professional perspective Identification of your strengths and your developmental needs
Planning	Determining where it is you want to be Identifying developmental goals and those actions needed and required to achieve your goals
Doing	Implementing your plan, experiencing the learning Bringing together and documenting the evidence of learning
Reflecting	Undertaking a review of your development through reflection Evaluating your achievements, making sense of them Identifying and discovering further developmental needs
Recording	Recording and storing the evidence associated with your achievements in relation to your planned goals

Source: adapted from Reed (2011) and Timmins and Duffy (2011).

Your university will provide you with guidance concerning how to complete the PDP; for example, you may be required to complete a new one for each term or for every module or course undertaken. A pro forma is usually made available for you to adhere to; you should check this out prior to commencing your PDP. There may be a requirement that you need to agree and sign off your PDP with your personal tutor.

Some advantages of using a PDP include:

- providing a sharper focus to your learning,
- helping to keep you motivated,
- helping you to understand how you learn and how you might improve performance,
- reducing stress from your learning as you develop into a consciously skilled thinker,
- generating awareness of how to apply learning to new challenges and situations,
- enhancing your reflective thinking skills,
- promoting greater confidence in the choices you make,
- being more articulate in discussing your skills, personal qualities and competencies with employers,
- becoming more confident and competent at problem solving.

SECTION SUMMARY

The professional portfolio is an essential component of your programme of study and will clearly show your experience, your achievements and how you have developed. Your professional portfolio will distinguish you from the competition. It provides examples of your unique strengths. Nurses need to provide evidence of their growth and achievement over time. The professional portfolio is a vehicle that helps you collect and present that evidence. Personal development plans are a key element of your professional portfolio and can help you to identify specific focused aspects of your learning.

PEARLS OF WISDOM

It takes much planning and hard work to weed out those unnecessary components of the professional portfolio and be able to promote positive feelings through it. You should be proud to show off your professional portfolio!

The structure and content of a professional portfolio

Preparing a portfolio may be a daunting experience for some people but there is help and guidance available. Your university may have already stated the structure and content of your professional portfolio, and you will need to determine if this is the case. Clark (2010b) notes that the structure may have been based on course learning outcomes or a formal learning contract may be in place between you and your mentor or supervisor. There may be strict rules about the portfolio particularly if it is going to be assessed as part of your programme of study. Other factors impacting on what is to go into the portfolio and how it is to be structured will include the format to be used.

Your professional portfolio is a visual and tangible way in which you can provide evidence of learning, and introduce yourself to interviewers and potential employers. In addition it will be needed, if, for example, you are seeking opportunities to join committees (at the university or elsewhere) or internal promotion or if you are changing your career. It can be used as evidence when you are undergoing performance review/appraisal. As a result of the power and potential of your portfolio you will need to give much thought to what you put into it. Figure 14.2 outlines some of the possible elements of the professional portfolio but, the content will be determined by its intended purpose.

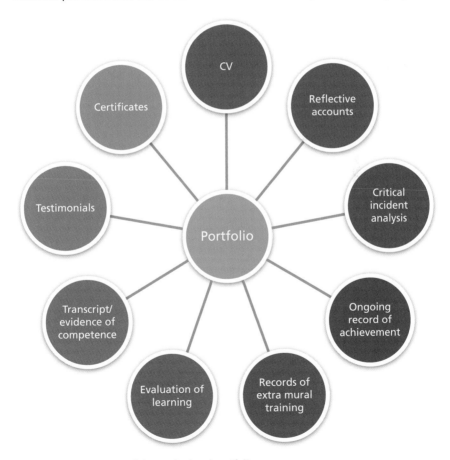

Figure 14.2 The content of the professional portfolio.

There are no hard-and-fast rules concerning what the portfolio should contain but the principles and processes are similar (Clark, 2010a): a profile is about capturing learning. The content should be tailored to meet your needs; therefore, if you are required to collect evidence concerning reflections on patient interaction as part of an assessed piece of work your portfolio must contain that evidence. The contents of the portfolio can be used to demonstrate that you are practising within, as well as understanding, the tenets enshrined in the NMC code of professional conduct (Nursing and Midwifery Council, 2008). For example, the code demands that you treat each person as an individual, so in your portfolio you can demonstrate the ways in which you have upheld that particular clause of the *Code*, addressing the moral and ethical issues that you may have faced to ensure individualised nursing care.

ACTIVITY 14.1

Before going any further, take some time to think about what should go into your portfolio. At the end of the chapter see if your list matches what has been discussed.

 Table of contents

This shows your reader the various sections and pages of your portfolio. Dividers should be used so as to clearly mark where one section ends and the other begins, section headings should be clear and follow a sequence. This helps the reader cross-refer and find their way around the portfolio.

 Introduction

The introduction will describe the structure of the portfolio and introduce you to the reader; this can be your profile accompanied by your goals, aims and aspirations. The whole document should be signposted throughout, showing how the many parts fit together to make the whole. Provide the reader with a sentence or two on the purpose of the portfolio and what they can expect to see in it.

You might be required (or you might want to) include a personal statement; this can resemble a personal mission statement. It is a statement of your personal philosophy, a short description of what is important to you, expressing points such as what you do or want to do, how you do it and why.

Curriculum vitae and work history

Including your CV is helpful as it gives the reader a picture of who you are and what you have done (the CV must include work history). Refer back to Chapter 1 and the brief discussion of CV content there. Some tips for CV writing can be found in Box 14.1.

Box 14.1 Some tips for CV writing

- Keep all fonts the same style, size and colour. Avoid writing your name in a font that is larger than that used in the rest of the CV. If you are using a header or footer, ensure the font is the same as the body of your CV.
- Present the information in chronological order, beginning with the most recent. Failure to do this means that your CV will read as if it is jumping all over the place. List education, experiences and activities in order.
- You should make use of strong action verbs when you are describing skills, responsibilities or accomplishments; be consistent. For example, use *developed* as opposed to *helped*, use *initiated* instead of *got involved*.
- Include any clinical experience you have had as a student. Be brief and don't forget to include any unique experiences. For example, if you spent time in a hospice or working with the homeless.
- Include details of your nursing elective if you have undertaken one.
- Proofread your CV and ensure you do not make any spelling errors. It might help to read the CV out loud. The spellchecker on your word processor will not flag up errors such as *week* instead of *weak* or *to* instead of *too*.
- You should not include any personal history, such as ethnicity, age, marital status or health.
- Be confident.

Personal/educational development certificates

These include school certificates (A levels), further education certificates (BTEC, qualifications and certificate framework: NVQ/SNVQ) and higher education degrees (BSc, BA). You should state what subjects the certificates (awards) are in and when you achieved them. Be sure to include factors such as the classification (i.e. merit, distinction). It is inappropriate to include other certificates you may have been awarded at school; for example, a swimming certificate.

In-house training courses (work-based)

In this section you should include and detail any in-house on-the-job training courses you have attended and passed. These can include any IT training (don't forget to include the level and, if appropriate, the application), moving and handling courses, vulnerable people courses, equality and diversity training and first aid training.

Self-analysis/feedback

This section will demonstrate to the reader your preferred learning style. If you have carried out a SWOT analysis (see Activity 14.2) and then put together a personal development plan or an action plan then include this as well. You may have used other self-analysis or feedback tools, such as personality inventories. The results of these should also be included.

ACTIVITY 14.2

SWOT stands for strengths, weaknesses, opportunities and threats. Undertake your own SWOT analysis using the template below.

Strengths	Weaknesses
☼ What skills or experience do you already possess?	☼ What areas of your development do you think you could improve on?
☼ Provide examples of how these skills have been used.	☼ What experience are you missing that you might need for your long-term nursing career?
☼ What is it that you already do well?	☼ What do you do badly?
☼ When others think of you, what do they see are your strengths?	☼ What should you avoid?
☼ Take time to think about these from your own perspective and the perspective of others.	☼ Do you have any weaknesses that your peers, friends or family think you have that you do not agree with?
☼ Don't be shy or hesitant; be realistic.	☼ If this is so, why do you think they may feel that?

Opportunities	Threats
☃ What activities and opportunities (human and material) are there available to help you in your learning and development?	☃ Take time to think about the obstacles that you face when getting involved in other activities.
☃ Consider the various interactions and contacts available to you (including those at university and on your practice placements). How will you ensure that you make best use of these?	☃ Are there any constraints imposed by other commitments; for example, level to which skills have developed, knowledge deficit or time?
☃ Look at your strengths and ask, will any of these lead to opportunities? You can also consider your weaknesses and ask yourself whether there is any opportunity to eliminate them.	☃ Do you think any of your weaknesses could genuinely jeopardise your opportunities while on your nurse education programme? If so, what are they?
	☃ Do you have any previous experiences of trying and failing when aiming to realise your goals and aspirations? How might this affect you? What learning can come from this?

 Assessments from other

These can include testimonials, thank-you cards and references. If these are to be included be sure that any testimonials and thank-you cards from patients and their families are afforded confidentiality. You can also include assessment feedback in this section.

Verification of learning

This evidence can be from your written work or the work you carry out in the practice setting. What have you learned from your life experiences that you have brought into your nursing programme?

Ongoing action plans, personal development plans

These should be in short format, outlining what you have achieved, your current key learning needs, your aspirations and your career intentions. Your personal tutor will help you compile your portfolio, but you will be expected to contribute in a meaningful way and take ownership of the professional portfolio. You should make photocopies of important documents and put the photocopies in the portfolio, but you should also have the originals available should verification be required. At all times you should work within the policy laid down by your university.

Clark (2010a) makes the very important point that it is not the number of pieces of evidence that matter, but their quality and relevance, with different types of evidence demonstrating different types of learning. As time progresses you will fill your portfolio with the evidence required that demonstrates your learning and your achievements.

Box 14.2 provides a summary of issues that should be considered when putting the professional portfolio together.

Box 14.2 Compiling the professional portfolio: issues to be considered

- Remember that this is a *professional* portfolio.
- Remember who the reader is.
- You should adhere to the guidelines issued by your university.
- Respect the rules of confidentiality.
- The portfolio should be legible and user-friendly (check grammar and spelling).
- Pages should be numbered.
- Make the most of cross-referencing as it can avoid repetition.
- Use appendices but be judicious (and be sure to label them).
- Provide signposting by using headings and subheadings.
- You may wish to compile a glossary of terms.
- Use a reference list to support the content where appropriate.
- Be selective with the evidence you provide: be clear and concise and scholarly in your approach.
- Try to ensure that each section links to the next rather than compartmentalising.

For a professional portfolio to be of value it should be well documented and organised. The portfolio should be:

 structured,

 representative,

 selective.

Structured

A structured portfolio will be organised, complete and innovative in its presentation. You may need to consider the following.

- Is my portfolio neat?
- Are the contents presented and displayed in an organised way?
- Do the contents reflect its intended purpose?

Representative

As well as ensuring that structure is appropriate, your portfolio should also be all-inclusive. The documentation included within the portfolio should represent the scope of your work. It should be representative across the programme and the various courses you have undertaken. Here are some questions for you think about.

- Does my professional portfolio represent the types and levels of courses that I have attended during my programme of study?
- Does my portfolio present a cross-section of my work as a student?

Selective

It is natural for those who are preparing a professional portfolio to want to document everything. However, depending on the purpose of the portfolio you must give careful attention to what goes into it and you must be selective. Think about conciseness and selectivity. If you fail to consider these issues you may fail to document your work in the most effective way. Limit the contents of your portfolio to what is required by the university reviewer, ensuring that you keep the purpose in mind.

SECTION SUMMARY

It is essential that you adhere to any guidelines provided by your university with regards to the structure and content of a professional portfolio. If the structure and the content have already been dictated then be sure you meet the minimum requirements.

As it develops the professional portfolio becomes a visual and tangible way for you to provide evidence of learning as well as a way for you to introduce yourself to others. As you progress in your career it may be used as evidence when you have your performance review/appraisal. As a result of this, what you put in it will need to be given much thought: remember that it is a *professional* portfolio.

Your profile should be about capturing learning as well as providing evidence of your development. There is scope for creativity and the content should be tailored to meet your own needs.

Portfolio format

Having put the portfolio together and structured in a way that is meaningful to you and the reader it needs to be presented in a manner that will show if off at its best: here we consider the format. You may have no choice with regards to the portfolio format as it may have already been dictated to you. Ensure that you check the guidelines issued to you. You can be as creative as you like: the portfolio lets you show what you have achieved and what can be achieved. Portfolio formats can vary considerably.

 I always thought that a portfolio was an upmarket word for a ring binder. *Miriam, first year student nurse*

Paper portfolio

The conventional way of presenting a portfolio, and what has been alluded to mostly throughout this chapter, is to use ring binders and paper. This is currently the most common format used and it is the simplest. The discussion has provided you with information concerning presentation. The conventional format is only one type: as technology advances other systems are available, such as an e-portfolio.

E-portfolios

These portfolios (also called digital portfolios) are usually commercially produced and act as an online electronic documentation and storage system. E-portfolios are useful as a green alternative to conventional paper portfolios and they can conveniently be e-mailed to lecturers or prospective employers for review. They are designed to provide evidence of learning and achievement and demonstrate both descriptive and reflective learning. They are a record of what the student thinks and has done and what others think of the student. Others, such as mentors and university lecturers, can access the e-portfolio.

What the e-portfolio records is closely aligned to the content to the undergraduate nursing programme being studied, including evidence of assessment and achievements (just as is required in the conventional way).

 I use the e-portfolio as a tool to aid me in my learning. It's easy to access where and when I want; I keep mine on my tablet. *Jaylee, second year student*

Those who are experienced with using computers and software packages can use animation and a variety of other multimedia effects to showcase achievements and act as appendices to their work. The e-portfolio can have these attributes:

- organised,
- searchable,
- transportable.

Just as there are disadvantages to using the conventional paper and binder portfolio so too are there disadvantages with e-portfolios. The main disadvantages are the level of IT proficiency needed. Students also need to have access to the Internet. Issues such as the security of content must also be given consideration as there is ample opportunity for invasion of privacy by someone other than the intended reader. The e-portfolio will allow you to include more content and samples of your work, but this will also mean that you will have to back-up your portfolio to keep it from being corrupted or lost due to a computer malfunction. An e-portfolio has the potential to take up a lot of digital storage space; therefore, in certain situations it may need to be put on either a CD or a flash drive. If you want to present your e-portfolio to your mentor or lecturer you will have to ensure that they are able to open and read the media you give them.

SECTION SUMMARY

The conventional way of putting together a portfolio is to use paper and a ring binder: this format is also the simplest. This approach is changing and the e-portfolio (or digital portfolio) is growing in popularity. Both formats have pros and cons and you should be aware of these.

Summary

You should not think that portfolio development ends when you have graduated, as it is never final (see Chapter 18). The portfolio (in whatever format) forms part of your ability to demonstrate your commitment to lifelong learning and currently it is your way of providing evidence that you are fully up to date with practice when you register and periodically re-register as a nurse with the NMC.

There are a variety of reasons why a professional portfolio is required. In essence a professional portfolio is a collection of wisely selected materials that document the competencies you have achieved and the various milestones met as you go through your undergraduate nurse education programme. The portfolio is developed over time and monitors your professional development. The portfolio is dynamic and fluid, changing as you progress, transforming as you do; your mentors and university staff will review it as you meet your personal, academic and professional goals.

 ## References

Benner, P. (1984) *From Novice to Expert. Excellence and Power in Clinical Nursing Practice.* Addison-Wesley, Menlo Park, CA

Clark, A.C. (2010a) How to compile a professional portfolio of practice 1: aims and learning outcomes. *Nursing Times* 106(41), 12–14

Clark, A.C. (2010b) How to compile a professional portfolio of practice 2: structure and building evidence. *Nursing Times* 106(42), 14–17

Coffey, A. (2005) The clinical learning portfolio: a practice development experience in gerontological nursing. *Journal of Clinical Nursing* 14(suppl. 8B), 75–83

Farrell, M. (2008) The purpose of portfolios. In Timmins, F. (ed.), *Making Sense of Portfolios. A Guide for Nursing Students.* Open University Press, Maidenhead, pp. 22–51

Nursing and Midwifery Council (2008) *The Code: Standards of Conduct, Performance and Ethics for Nurses and Midwives.* Nursing and Midwifery Council, London

Nursing and Midwifery Council (2010) *Standards for Pre registration Nursing Education.* http://standards.nmc-uk.org/PublishedDocuments/Standards%20for%20pre-registration%20nursing%20education%2016082010.pdf

Nursing and Midwifery Council (2011) *The Prep Handbook.* www.nmc-uk.org/Documents/Standards/NMC_Prep-handbook_2011.pdf

Quality Assurance Agency for Higher Education (2009) *Personal Development Planning: Guidance for Institutional Policy and Practice in Higher Education.* www.qaa.ac.uk/Publications/InformationAndGuidance/Documents/PDPguide.pdf

Reed, S. (2011) *Successful Professional Portfolios for Nursing Students.* Learning Matters, Exeter

Scholes, J., Webb, C., Gray, M., Endacott, R., Miller, C., Jasper, M. And McMullan, M. (2004) Making portfolios work in practice. *Journal of Advanced Nursing* 46(6), 595–603

Timmins, F. and Duffy, A. (2011) *Writing your Nursing Portfolio. A Step by Step Guide.* Open University Press, Maidenhead

Twadell, J. and Johnson, J. (2007) A time for nursing portfolios: a tool for career development. *Advances in Neonatal Nursing* 7(3), 146–50

 ## Resources

Campaign for Learning

www.campaign-for-learning.org.uk/cfl/index.asp

The Campaign for Learning is working towards a society where learning is at the heart of social inclusion. A variety of helpful and interesting resources.

E-portfolio Portal

www.danwilton.com/eportfolios/

This website provides a resource to assist you in gaining knowledge around the concepts of e-portfolios.

Mind Tools

www.mindtools.com/

A site designed to help you learn the practical, straightforward skills you need to excel in your career. Hints and tips that will help you develop and understand how you learn best.

Skills for Study

www.palgrave.com/skills4study/index.asp

This is a free resource and is packed full of practical advice to help you study more effectively at university.

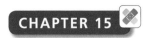

CHAPTER 15

 # Records and Record Keeping

WHAT THIS CHAPTER CONTAINS

- Information on documentation and record keeping
- A discussion about the reasons why records are kept
- An overview of the principles of good record keeping
- A discussion of your role in the maintenance and safety of records

Good record keeping is a fundamental aspect of nursing practice, it is a vital component associated with the provision of safe and effective nursing care. Record keeping should not be viewed as an optional extra to be fitted in if circumstances allow: it is a part of good clinical care. The importance of keeping accurate records cannot be underestimated; it is an integral aspect of your role.

The nursing record is only of any value if it is accurate, timely and comprehensive. Record keeping that falls below this standard is of little value. Good record keeping is essential if the nurse is to provide safe and effective care. It helps to protect the welfare of the people in your care.

 ## Documentation

Records and record keeping that comply with the guidance provided by the NMC (Nursing and Midwifery Council, 2009) will enable you to validate and provide:

- a full description of the assessment and the care planned and given to people,
- appropriate information about the people being cared for at any given time and what you did in responding to their needs,
- confirmation that you have understood and satisfied your duty of care, that you have taken all reasonable steps to care for the person and that the actions you have taken or those you have decided to omit have not compromised the person's safety in any way,
- a record of any arrangement you have made for care that is to continue with another healthcare provider (allowing nurses and other care providers to communicate about the care given).

The Student Nurse Toolkit: An Essential Guide for Surviving Your Course, First Edition. Ian Peate.
© 2013 John Wiley & Sons, Ltd. Published 2013 by John Wiley & Sons, Ltd.

There will be local policies in place guiding the nurse with respect to records and record keeping. Even though the NMC (Nursing and Midwifery Council, 2009) provides guidance, it does not determine the content, and so there is no rigid framework provided for the content of records or record keeping. What to include and exclude and the format used for a patient's records and other documents is left to the accountable practitioner, and relies on professional judgement.

Any investigations into complaints (internally or externally) about care will consider and use the patient's documents and records as evidence, and as such high-quality record keeping is crucial. A number of official bodies can make investigations as a result of complaints and can include:

- a hospital,
- a care home,
- the NMC,
- Care Quality Commission (and other health and social care regulators),
- a court of law,
- the police.

A court of law will be of the opinion that if care has not been recorded then it has not been given.

When Fitness to Practice Committees are investigating complaints made about nurses the NMC may also request records, including:

- care plans,
- diaries,
- anything making reference to the patient.

In every health and social care setting you will come across lots of different types of documentation; for example, charts, forms and case notes. All hospitals, care homes and community nursing services will have the same basic types of document. There will, however, be variations on the different themes, matching them to meet local needs.

ACTIVITY 15.1

Make a list of the various types of documentation you have seen when you have been working in various health and social care settings.

Your list may have run on for pages and pages as there is so much documentation used in the various sectors. Common types of documents that you will have seen and used include the following:

- nursing assessment sheets,
- nursing care plans,
- observation charts,
- fluid balance charts,
- risk-assessment sheets,
- medication charts,
- incident forms.

Box 15.1 lists the types of records covered by the Department of Health (2006a) code of practice concerning records management.

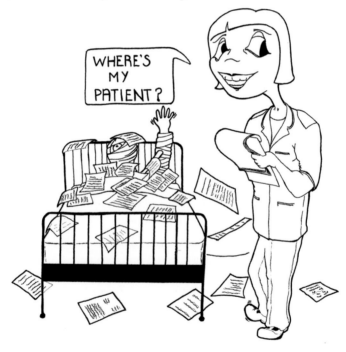

Box 15.1 Types of records covered by the Department of Health's *Code of Practice*

- Patient health records (electronic or paper-based, including those concerning all specialties, and GP medical records)
- Records of private patients seen on NHS premises
- Accident and emergency, birth and all other registers

- Theatre registers and minor operations (and other related) registers
- Administrative records (including, for example, personnel, estates, financial and accounting records, notes associated with complaint-handling)
- X-ray and imaging reports, output and images, photographs, slides, and other images, microform (i.e. microfiche/microfilm), audio and video tapes, cassettes, CD-ROM, memory sticks, e-mails
- Computerised records, scanned records
- Text messages (both outgoing from the NHS and incoming responses from the patient)

Source: Department of Health (2006a).

 ## Definitions

The term documentation is used to mean any written or electronically generated information about a patient that describes the care or services they have been provided with. Health records can be paper documents or electronic documents; for example, electronic medical records, faxes, e-mails, audio or video tapes and images. Through documentation, nurses communicate their observations, decisions, actions and outcomes of these actions for the people they care for. Documentation should be an accurate account of what occurred and when it occurred.

According to the Department of Health (2010) a care record is:

> any paper or electronic-based record which contains information or personal data pertaining to people's care.

The Data Protection Act 1998 defines a health record as:

> consisting of information about the physical or mental health or condition of an identifiable individual made by or on behalf of a health professional in connection with the care of that individual.

SECTION SUMMARY

There are a number of definitions available for what is meant by documentation or a healthcare record. All documentation pertaining to a patient and their health can be seen as a patient record, and a court of law may be of the opinion that if care has not been recorded then you have not provided it.

> " I was (and I suppose still am to some respects) really nervous with the record keeping thing. I was anxious that I was not putting enough info in and everyone kept saying 'the care plan can be used in court so get it right'. I chilled out and now my entries are precise and succinct after my mentor said 'keep it relevant; no gossip'. *Dianne, third year student* "

Reasons for documentation

Clear, relevant and accurate documentation is an essential component of nurses' accountability and provides a way for nurses to account for their actions and omissions. High-quality documentation is therefore critical. The healthcare record is not a legal document, but a tool permitting the healthcare team to:

- communicate effectively,
- deliver appropriate, individualised, patient-centred care,
- evaluate the progress and health outcomes of patients,
- retain the integrity of health information over time.

However, the healthcare record can be admitted as evidence, if relevant, in legal proceedings.

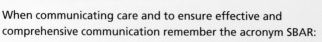

PEARLS OF WISDOM

When communicating care and to ensure effective and comprehensive communication remember the acronym SBAR:

S is for situation (identify the person and the reason for admission)

B is for background (provide a brief and significant history, including tests or treatments completed)

A is for assessment (describe the person's current condition)

R is for recommendation (discuss the person's plan of care)

Box 15.2 provides details concerning record keeping as outlined in the NMC code of professional conduct (Nursing and Midwifery Council, 2008).

Box 15.2 Guidance for nurses for keeping clear and accurate records

- You must keep clear and accurate records of the discussions you have, the assessments you make, the treatment and medicines you give and how effective these have been.
- You must complete records as soon as possible after an event has occurred.

- ℧ You must not tamper with original records in any way.
- ℧ You must ensure any entries you make in someone's paper records are clearly and legibly signed, dated and timed.
- ℧ You must ensure any entries you make in someone's records are clearly attributable to you.
- ℧ You must ensure all records are kept securely.

Source: Nursing and Midwifery Council (2009).

Putting together the healthcare record requires you to provide comprehensive, accurate, high-quality documentation. There is a variety of reasons why nurses and other healthcare professionals are required to document patient care, their activity or other events.

 ## To facilitate communication

When nurses are documenting they are communicating with other nurses and care providers with details about their assessments concerning the health status of their patient, nursing interventions that are carried out and the outcomes of these interventions. Documenting this information reinforces the aim that the person will receive consistent and informed care or service provision; it enables a seamless approach. Systematic, thorough and accurate documentation reduces the potential for miscommunication and errors. Most documentation is usually carried out by nurses and other care providers; there are situations however, when the client and family may document observations or care provided to communicate this information with members of the healthcare team.

 ## To promote good nursing care

Documentation encourages nurses to assess patient progress and establish which interventions are effective and which are ineffective, and to identify and document changes to the plan of care as required. Nurses can use outcome information or information from a critical incident to reflect on their practice and make any changes needed based on evidence.

 ## To meet professional and legal standards

Documentation has the potential to demonstrate (provide evidence) that, within the nurse–patient relationship, the nurse has applied nursing knowledge, skills and judgement according to professional standards (those outlined in the *Code*; Nursing and Midwifery Council, 2008). The nurse's documentation can be called as evidence in legal proceedings such as lawsuits, coroners' inquests and disciplinary hearings through professional regulatory bodies (the NMC). In a court of law, the person's health record acts as the legal record of the care or service provided.

Nursing care and the documentation of that care will be measured according to the standard of a reasonable nurse with similar education and experience in a similar situation.

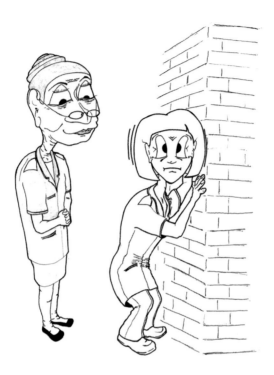

SECTION SUMMARY

The reasons for keeping documentation vary. The key purpose is to communicate about the person's health and well-being and to deliver appropriate, individualised, patient-centred care. Whereas it is acknowledged that the healthcare record is not a legal document, it can to be admitted as evidence, if relevant, in legal proceedings.

The principles of good record keeping

Continuity of care includes the principle that any other nurse or healthcare worker (for example, student or healthcare assistant) should be able to pick up a care plan, a chart or a person's notes and understand the status of that individual's condition and care. The provision of high-quality care is a team effort and each person's individual needs must be clearly communicated to all members of that team. Where appropriate, the person in your care, or their carer, should be involved in the record-keeping process.

Below are some of the principles involved, providing you with a clear direction for producing and maintaining high-quality, meaningful documentation.

 ## Document fact not fiction

Fact is what you have seen, heard or done in relation to the patient's care and condition. This is what you should be documenting. You should avoid non-committal documentation – for example, the use of words such as 'appears' or 'seems' – as these do not represent factual documentation. An extension of this principle is that you should write healthcare records objectively. Irrespective of where the nurse is recording information, be it in the nursing notes, on an incident form or as part of a statement, documentation should always remain factual and objective, avoiding subjectivity or emotion.

 ## Document all relevant information

What constitutes relevant information will be dictated by consideration of the individual circumstances of each patient. Your documentation should be made with respect to the total condition of the patient (a holistic approach), not just a clinical specialty. You should, in particular, document any change in the condition of the patient and who was notified of such a change. The use of early warning systems (see Chapter 5) demands that you make known to whom you have reported any deterioration in condition. Nurses should also document whether the patient's condition has remained unchanged during their shift, as responsibility for the patient is handed over with each change of shift.

Changes in condition should always be documented in the appropriate notes or on the relevant chart, as well as any intentional omissions of a specific treatment or procedure and why it was omitted. If a record is not made it may be assumed that the treatment or procedure was simply overlooked or forgotten.

Documentation should be made with total clarity. When documenting this you should ensure that you include a precise record of what aspect of the patient's condition was of concern, who was informed of the person's condition, exactly what they were told, when and the response received.

ACTIVITY 15.2

A patient is prescribed 250 mcg of digoxin. Prior to giving the medication you take the patient's pulse for a full minute and it is 56 beats per minute. Working with your supervisor the decision is given to omit the drug. How would you document that omission? What information would you need to include in the documentation? How would you care for the patient who was expecting to receive the dose of digoxin? Who else needs to be informed? Give a rationale for your responses.

 Document contemporaneously

This means documenting at the same period of time (contemporary). Record entries should be made in the person's notes as soon as possible after the events have occurred. Each entry should be dated and the time included, not forgetting a signature, printed name and designation (local policy will determine protocol). This approach makes clear when the record was made and by whom; documentation in this respect is more reliable. It is unacceptable to pre-date or pre-time any entry made in the person's notes, records or charts. When medication is given or an observation is made the time the drug is given and the time the observation was made should be recorded on the appropriate charts.

ACTIVITY 15.3

You might be required to rely on your records to support your actions, clinical decision making and the care that you gave to a patient many years after the event took place. This activity is intended to show how we should not take our record keeping for granted.
a Make a note of what you were doing this time last week.

b Can you recall what you were doing at this time last month?

c Can you remember what you were doing on this date last year?

d Try now and remember what you were doing 4 years ago....

 ## Preserve the integrity of the document

This means all that has been recorded in a person's notes should be preserved, even if errors have been made. You should never attempt to delete or alter any errors. If any attempt is made to alter any entry then it may be interpreted as an attempt to mislead or cover up. The error should be left so that it is legible. Local policy will dictate how this is to be managed. You may be required to put a single line through the error, and to date, sign and write your name next to the mistake. The correct entry should be made next to the error, on the next line or in the next column. Do not leave any space in the documentation or breaks in the narrative; this prevents any information being added after the event. To avoid misinterpretation when mistakes or errors are made (and they do occur) they should be clearly identified as such.

 ## Litigation

Potential litigation is an issue that we would probably rather not consider; however, a patient record may form the basis for litigation. When litigation has been instigated and records are inspected an expert witness who is working for the complainant will review them. It is the role of the expert witness to give an opinion on the quality and appropriateness of the care provided and this will be deduced from the records available. The law expects a nurse to act as a reasonable nurse with the same level of training and experience would act in a similar situation. The nursing record will be scrutinised line by line, in part to ascertain whether this legal standard has been met. The nurse's best defence is an accurate nursing record. See also Chapter 16, which concerns legal issues.

Failure to comply with guidance provided by the NMC (Nursing and Midwifery Council, 2009) may lead to you being called to account for your actions or omissions, and charges may be made against you as a result of inadequate or falsified documentation. Questions may be raised about your ability to practise in a competent manner. Errors do occur in record keeping and Box 15.3 highlights some of these.

Box 15.3 Some errors made in record keeping

- ☼ Time omitted
- ☼ Handwriting that is impossible to read, illegible
- ☼ Abbreviations that are vague/unclear
- ☼ Use of correction fluid to conceal errors
- ☼ No signature
- ☼ Errors, specifically concerning dates
- ☼ Gaps in completing the record
- ☼ Notes completed by a person who did not care for the patient
- ☼ Mistakes relating to patient's name, date of birth and address
- ☼ Unprofessional, sarcastic terminology, e.g. 'a moody person'
- ☼ Meaningless expressions, e.g. 'pleasant person'
- ☼ Opinion and facts combined
- ☼ Subjective as opposed to objective comments, e.g. 'had a good day'
- ☼ Using initials in records (a full signature should be used with the nurse's name written alongside it)

Source: adapted from Dimond (2011).

ACTIVITY 15.4

Select two sets of hand-held nursing records at random (try to choose those in which you have recently made entries).
Using the NMC's guidance on the principles of good record keeping (Nursing and Midwifery Council, 2009), complete an audit of these records.
Criteria you might want to focus on:
- ☼ are all the entries legible?

- ☼ have they all been dated and timed?

- ☼ did you print your name and job title alongside the initial entry (and other carers, too)?

- ☼ has black, indelible ink been used throughout?

Good documentation includes the following.

- Be accurate. For example, do not use vague terms such as 'good urine output'. How many millilitres are 'good?' Document the amount that has been voided, at what time and what the urine looked like. Avoid terms like 'reasonable' or 'adequate'. They are vague and they mean little.
- Document objective information. Document only what you see, feel, smell and hear. If you are writing what someone else observed, then this should be clearly reflected in the notes. You may quote the patient, but be sure to indicate that as such. For example, 'My back hurts', and note it as per patient, including the use of inverted commas. Do not note, 'patient fell', if you find a patient on the floor. Although this is more than likely what occurred, unless you saw it happen you cannot be sure. Document, 'patient found on the floor' and any other relevant information.
- Document as soon as possible after care has been provided. Never document medications before they are administered, or care episodes or procedures before they are performed.
- Write legibly. Errors are more likely to occur if others cannot read your writing. Write in black, indelible ink.
- Use only approved abbreviations. If unsure as to what the abbreviation may mean then you must seek advice, spelling the words out. Taking shortcuts can have dire implications for the people you care for.

PEARLS OF WISDOM

Use the ELBOW rule when making notes.

No **e**rasions (of any kind)

No **l**eaves (pages) pulled out or removed

No **b**lank spaces (draw a line across any blank space)

No **o**verwriting (use the formal method of amendments)

No **w**riting in margins, as this is only used for the time and date of the entry

SECTION SUMMARY

The NMC has issued guidance concerning record keeping. When nurses adhere to the principles of good documentation then high-quality care will ensue. Care documented must be accurate and objective and it should be documented as soon as possible after a care episode.

The use of abbreviations, acronyms and symbols

Effective record keeping is the hallmark of a skilled, competent, confident and safe practitioner and can result in effective communication. However, the message being communicated will only be as good as the person who is recording the information. Abbreviations that are used in one care area may not mean the same in another. It must be remembered that other healthcare workers will be depending on the information contained in the records that you make and, as a result of what you have documented (including the use of abbreviations and acronyms), may act on it. The use of abbreviations, symbols or acronyms can be an efficient form of documentation if their meaning is well understood by everyone. Abbreviations and symbols that are obscure, obsolete, poorly defined or have multiple meanings have the potential to lead to errors, cause confusion and waste people's time.

The use of abbreviations and acronyms in healthcare has become an international patient safety issue. There are a number of common problems and these include ambiguous, unfamiliar and look-alike abbreviations as well as acronyms leading to misinterpretation and healthcare errors.

Abbreviations are often used to save time. For example, in some care areas the abbreviations T for temperature, BP for blood pressure, P for pulse and R for respiration are used routinely; it could be suggested that if healthcare workers did not use abbreviations in their work then even more time would be needed for record keeping. If abbreviations are used then it is recommended that an organisation compile a list of approved abbreviations and acceptable symbols with the intention of reducing the risk of error, misinterpretation and misunderstanding.

ACTIVITY 15.5

Make a list of the abbreviations that are common in your daily practice. Take some time and think, can any of them be interpreted in more than one way?

In the examples below think about how they may be interpreted.

- IUD_____
- SB_____
- PROM_____
- CPD_____
- POM_____

You may be putting the people you care for at risk by using abbreviations. Nurses communicate in many ways, especially when documenting patient information. However, if what you write does not communicate a clear message, then you have failed in your professional and legal responsibilities. When documenting, it is essential that you do not put your patient's health and well-being at risk because of the methods you use for the task, including the use of abbreviations. Indiscriminately using abbreviations can be very dangerous and should be avoided as they can be a total mystery to the reader and they are easily confused. If you are going to use abbreviations:

 exercise much care and be extremely careful,

 use them as little as possible,

 stay within the approved abbreviation list,

 print them carefully,

 use the appropriate capitalisation and full stops,

 do not invent new abbreviations.

PEARLS OF WISDOM

If you are reading abbreviations and you do not know what the abbreviation means, do not guess their meaning. Seek clarification from the writer.

> During handover the nurse in charge said that one of the patients was NPO. I had never heard of this, and I was too shy to ask in front of everyone. When I had a moment alone with my mentor I asked him what it was she meant and he said he didn't know. I plucked up courage and asked the sister and she tutted at me, saying 'anyone knows it means nil per oral'. I still didn't understand and at that point my mentor stepped in and he said he didn't know what it meant, it meant nil by mouth. NPO is a phrase they use in the States; she had just come back from working over there. Lesson learned: 'when in doubt, shout'.
> *Willkie, third year student*

Prior to starting to write an abbreviation, think about it. Consider whether it is in the patient's best interest: is it the best use of everyone's time and is it the best way for you to discharge your professional duties? If you do not know what an abbreviation means, then the writer has not communicated effectively. You can guess at what is trying to be said but you may guess incorrectly and put the health and well-being of the people in your care in serious jeopardy.

Maintaining the safety of records

The registered nurse is professionally accountable for any duties that they choose to delegate to any other member of the interprofessional healthcare team, such as the student nurse. Delegation of duties can include the delegation of record keeping to pre-registration nursing students. As a student you must be supervised appropriately and you must demonstrate that you are capable of carrying out the task. The registered nurse should countersign any entry in the notes, care plans and other documents demonstrating their professional accountability for the consequences of such an entry.

You are required to keep up to date with and to adhere to relevant legislation, case law, and national and local policies relating to information and record keeping.

 ## Confidentiality and disclosure

Currently, records are kept in the place where the person receives their care. Usually, these institutions can only share information from the person's records by letter, e-mail, fax or telephone. Being aware of the legal requirements and other guidance concerning confidentiality, which can help to ensure that your practice is in line with national and local policies. Local and national rules governing confidentiality in respect of the supply and use of data for secondary purposes must be followed and this is the case when using records for research purposes. Chapter 6 addresses some issues associated with confidentiality.

You must never discuss the people in your care in places where you might be overheard. Furthermore, do not leave records, either on paper or on a computer screen, where unauthorised staff or members of the public could see them.

Any information that can identify a person who you are caring for must never be used or disclosed for reasons other than healthcare without the person's clear consent. There are times, however, when you can release this information; for example, if the law requires it or when there is a greater public interest. You are allowed to disclose information under common law if it will help to prevent, detect, investigate or punish serious crime or if it will prevent abuse or serious harm to others.

 ## Access

People for whom you care should be informed that information on their health records might be seen by other people or agencies involved in their care. The aim of the Access to Medical Reports Act 1988 is to allow individuals to see medical reports written about them.

People in your care have a right to ask to see their own health records; if this happens you need to be aware of your local policy and be able to explain it to the person if they request access to their record. The patient may view the report by obtaining a photocopy, or by attending the organisation to read the report without taking a copy away. The patient has a right to view the report from the time it is written. However, in certain circumstances the person may be prohibited from viewing all or part of the report if:

- in the opinion of the doctor, viewing the report may cause serious harm to the physical or mental health of the patient; or
- access to the report would disclose third-party information when that third party has not consented to the disclosure (Department of Health, 2010).

Patients have the right to ask for any of their information to be withheld from you or other health professionals and you must respect that right unless there is concern that by withholding such information this would cause serious harm to that person or others.

If you are experiencing any problems relating to access or record keeping – for example, missing records or problems accessing records – and you are unable to resolve the problem, you should report the matter to a person in authority. Ensure that you keep a record detailing this report.

You must never retrieve the records of any person, or their family, to find out personal information that is not relevant to their care.

 ## Security and information systems

Within the various practice placements you attend there will be a number of information tools and systems available you. You should be aware of and appreciate how to use them.

If you are issued with smartcards or passwords to access information systems they must not be shared. Do not leave systems open to access by others when you have finished using them: shut them down as per policy. Ensure that you use the various systems appropriately, particularly in relation to confidentiality.

 A bigwig doctor asked me to leave the screen open for him to look at some blood results. I politely refused and boy was he hacked off, but I knew that giving passwords or leaving systems open was a no no. I used this situation for one of my reflective pieces at uni.
Marty, second year student

 ## Safe disposal of records

All organisations must have in place disposal arrangements for the destruction, archiving and closure of records and procedures that will prevent unnecessary copying of information (Department of Health, 2006a). Records (regardless of the medium) may be retained for longer than the minimum period. However, records should not ordinarily be retained for more than 30 years (Department of Health, 2006b). How long records should be kept will depend on the type of record, as different types will be kept for different periods of time. In England the Department of Health has produced guidance on disposal and retention of records (Department of Health, 2006a, 2006b).

Hospital records are usually held for a minimum of 8 years after the conclusion of treatment but there are lots of exceptions, such as children and young people, maternity records and mental health records (see Table 15.1). The Department of Health guidance addresses a great number of different types of health records and specifies the length of time they should be kept (this is called the minimum retention period). The guidance applies regardless of how the records are held, for example:

- paper records,
- electronic records,
- images,
- sound.

Table 15.1 Examples of health records and their minimum retention periods

Type of record	Details
GP records	Until 10 years after the patient's death or after the patient has permanently left the country, unless they remain in the European Union Electronic patient records must not be destroyed or deleted for the foreseeable future
Vaccination records	Children and young people: until the patient is 25 (or 26 if they are 17 when treatment ends) Other vaccination records: 10 years after treatment ends
Dental, ophthalmic and auditory screening records	Community records: - Adults: 11 years - Children: 11 years or until the patient is 25, whichever is longer Hospital records: - Adults: 8 years - Children: until the patient is 25 (or 26 if they are 17 when treatment ends) or, if sooner, 8 years after their death
Children and young people	All types of records: - Until the patient is 25 (or 26 if they are 17 when treatment ends) or, if sooner, 8 years after their death - If a child's illness or death could be relevant to an adult condition or have genetic implications for their family, records may be kept for longer
Maternity records (including obstetric and midwifery records)	25 years after the birth of the last child
Records relating to people with a mental disorder (within the meaning of any mental health act)	20 years after the last contact between the patient and any healthcare professional or, if sooner, 8 years after the patient's death

Source: Department of Health (2006b).

This guidance also applies to records about patients treated on behalf of the NHS in the private healthcare sector.

SECTION SUMMARY

Each nurse has a responsibility to ensure that any record is stored safely and disposed of in the most appropriate way; guidance has been issued to help ensure that this happens. People expect that their records will be treated with respect and this includes an expectation that they will be kept confidential and the contents only used for the purpose for which they were originally intended.

 ## Summary

The use of records is another method of communication and you must ensure that you are communicating effectively. Guidance has been produced by the NMC with regard to record keeping and this should be adhered to so that the person being cared for is safe.

The importance of keeping accurate records should never be underestimated; it is an essential aspect of the role and function of the nurse. The nursing record will only be of any value if it is accurate, timely and comprehensive. Record keeping that falls below this standard is of little value and may be deemed misconduct.

Local and national policy and protocol dictate how records are to be managed and this includes their content, safety and disposal. The term documentation means any written or electronically generated information about a patient that describes the care or services they have been provided with. Through documentation, nurses communicate their observations, decisions and actions. Documentation should be an accurate account of what occurred and when it occurred and is only as good as the people who complete it.

 ## References

Department of Health (2006a) *Records Management: NHS Code of Practice (Part 1)*. Department of Health, London

Department of Health (2006b) *Records Management: NHS Code of Practice (Part 2)*. Department of Health, London

Department of Health (2010) *Essence of Care 2010: Benchmarks for Record Keeping*. Department of Health, London

Dimond, B. (2011) *Legal Aspects of Nursing*, 6th edn. Pearson, Colchester

Nursing and Midwifery Council (2008) *The Code: Standards of Conduct, Performance and Ethics for Nurses and Midwives*. Nursing and Midwifery Council, London

Nursing and Midwifery Council (2009) *Record Keeping. Guidance for Nurses and Midwives*. www.nmc-uk.org/Documents/NMC-Publications/NMC-Record-Keeping-Guidance.pdf

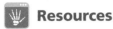

Resources

Advanced Nursing Practice Toolkit

www.advancedpractice.scot.nhs.uk/

The Advanced Nursing Practice Toolkit is a UK-wide repository for consistent, credible and helpful resources relating to advanced practice. It supports ongoing work across the sector to enhance understanding of this role, benchmarking of this level of practice and its application to specific roles across clinical practice, research, education and leadership.

Information Commissioner's Office

www.ico.gov.uk/for_organisations/data_protection.aspx

The Information Commissioner's Office is the UK's independent authority for upholding information rights in the public interest, promoting openness by public bodies and data privacy for individuals.

Scottish Information Commissioner

www.itspublicknowledge.info/home/ScottishInformationCommissioner.asp

The Scottish Information Commissioner is a public official appointed by Her Majesty the Queen on the nomination of the Scottish Parliament. The Commissioner is responsible for enforcing and promoting Scotland's freedom of information laws.

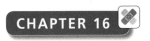 Protocols, Policies and Legal Matters

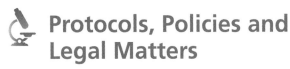

WHAT THIS CHAPTER CONTAINS

- An overview of nursing protocols and policies
- A discussion of a duty of care
- An outline of clinical negligence
- An overview of consent

This chapter provides a brief overview of some of the legal issues in nursing. The law impacts on every aspect of the role and function of the nurse and the discussion in this chapter is only an introduction. As you work through your programme of study you will learn and understand more about the law and how you must work within it. Protocols and policies also feature highly in the daily life of the nurse. Their status and use are described in this chapter.

Protocols and policies

Protocols

The terms protocol and policy are often used interchangeably. Nursing protocols are designed to help nurses react to clinical situations in a safe and appropriate manner with little or no guidance from colleagues. Protocols represent the framework for the management of a specific disorder or clinical situation, whereas the procedures that complement a specific protocol represent the many detailed steps for implementing that protocol.

The Working in Partnership Programme (2006) defines a protocol as an agreed framework outlining the care that will be provided to patients in a designated area of practice. There is a strict sequence of activities to be adhered to when a protocol is being used.

The Student Nurse Toolkit: An Essential Guide for Surviving Your Course, First Edition. Ian Peate.
© 2013 John Wiley & Sons, Ltd. Published 2013 by John Wiley & Sons, Ltd.

Those who are required to follow a protocol should easily understand it. Those working with a protocol should be able to assess whether they have the appropriate education and training and are competent to undertake the work. Protocols are an agreement (between a group of key stakeholders) to a particular sequence of activities, which can assist nurses in responding consistently in a complex area of clinical practice. Procedures are written when a task is highly technical and dependent on an exact order of events, or to support other healthcare staff (for example, a healthcare assistant) to develop competencies. A nursing protocol is usually divided into three parts:

- the first part defines the condition in detail,
- the second part describes the actual nursing plan (for example, drug and non-drug treatments, counselling, follow-up and referral),
- the final part lists the evidence base (the scientific references) that provide justification for the care plan.

Box 16.1 provides the details associated with a protocol.

Box 16.1 Details associated with a protocol

- Title page
  - Name of protocol
  - Reference number
  - Box for authors names
  - Date written
  - Date ratified
  - Review date
  - Name of reviewers
- Policy statement
- Rationale
- Criteria for performing the role
- Expectations of staff performing the role
- Protocols, guidelines and relevant paperwork
- Training requirements, expectations
- Competency statements
- Evidence and references (inclusive of references with other relevant Trust policies)
- Other appendices
- Review date

Protocols describe why, where, when and by whom care is given as opposed to how a specific procedure is to be performed. Clinical guidelines and clinical pathways are usually the tools that are used to specify how a procedure is to be performed and can help the nurse and others in the multidisciplinary team to making research- or evidence-based decisions about care in particular situations (Open Clinical, 2011). The advantages and disadvantages of clinical protocols can be seen in Table 16.1.

Table 16.1 Some advantages and disadvantages of clinical protocols

Advantages	Disadvantages
Provide a framework for a complex, specialised sequence of activities	Have the potential to stifle individual care management
Offer increased autonomy with a focus to shape future work	May cut the need for regulated staff
Ensure consensus within the primary care team	Require regular review
Can provide legal protection	Compliance may be challenging
Identify training needs	Can hinder clinical discretion
May facilitate change	

Source: adapted from Working in Partnership Programme (2006).

ACTIVITY 16.1

When you are next on placement retrieve three nursing protocols and consider their content with respect to the advantages and disadvantages in Table 16.1. How closely do they match?

A good protocol will detail clearly lines of accountability and provide reference to specific criteria. The protocol should be clear, brief and match professional guidelines. It will provide the reasons for the development of the protocol; the objectives should be stated clearly. Its intended use and applicability should be presented in an unambiguous manner. The health professionals and patients for whom the protocol is intended need to be identified. Details of any requirements for the application of the protocol will be included.

Clear, unambiguous language readily understood by all parties should be used. Any abbreviations must be written in full when used for the first time, with the subsequent abbreviation in parentheses. Accurate references to relevant national or local clinical guidelines or pathways should feature.

 ## Policies

Policies can be defined as purposeful plans of action that are directed towards a risk or an issue of concern (Sudduth, 2008). Friedman (2007) notes that a policy is what

you do; it is not what you write. Policies should be evidence-based wherever possible in terms of making the case for change and in evaluating their own effectiveness.

A policy is a specific statement of principles/guiding actions providing a basis for consistent decision making and resource allocation, whereas a procedure is a series of steps that are followed in regular order, taken to implement a policy. Procedures can usually be mapped using a flow chart. A guideline is a set of systematically developed standards or rules assisting in the decision about how to apply the policy or appropriate management of specific conditions. Guidelines are usually used to underpin a policy.

Collins and Patel (2009) suggest that policies in acute hospitals should be considered primarily as operational tools. They must be a concise and clearly understandable resource providing support and direction to staff, patients and the public.

Most healthcare providers have a broad network of policies extending across a range of clinical activities, including procedures to be undertaken by healthcare professionals to achieve a high standard of care. Just as protocols are developed by a group of stakeholders, this is also the case for policy development. Figure 16.1 provides a diagrammatic representation of the policy development process.

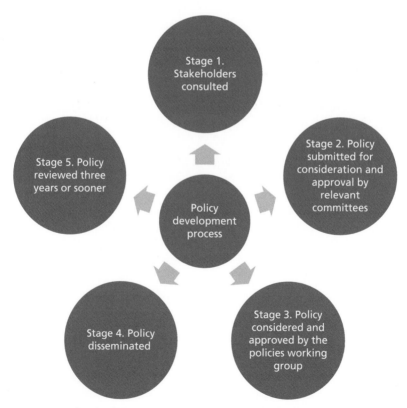

Figure 16.1 Policy development process. *Source*: adapted from Collins and Patel (2009).

Protocols and policies are there to help nurses provide safe and effective care, they can help to alleviate risk or harm to the people you care for. They are evidence based and should not be deviated from unless the patient's condition dictates; the nurse must be able to account for the deviation.

Duty of care

There are many reasons why nurses may fail to adhere to protocols or fail to use policies and procedures. However, regardless of these reasons a nurse is expected to adhere to a high standard of care that refers to the expected procedures, tasks and risk assessment required in the everyday working environment. When a nurse fails to meet the standard of care, their actions (or omissions) can put people at risk. The standard is set by the NMC through its code of professional conduct (Nursing and Midwifery Council, 2008).

ACTIVITY 16.2

Go to this page on the NMC website (www.nmc-uk.org/Hearings/Hearings-and-outcomes/), where you will find details about upcoming and completed hearings. The NMC publish information about all orders made by the committee panels and the reasons for those orders, and this includes the identity of the nurses and midwives concerned.

The NMC releases details of nurses and midwives affected by panel decisions to employers and the public. Names of nurses and midwives who have been referred to the NMC are not published until the case is referred to the Conduct and Competence or Health Committee. Cases that the Investigating Committee panel consider and then close are never published.

If a nurse fails to meet the standard of care, there may be an allegation of misconduct. The consequences for misconduct in a profession as important as nursing can be very extreme. As well as potentially harming or jeopardising the life of a patient, nurses can lose their job if misconduct is proven; they may also be named in legal cases and can even face criminal penalties. These consequences vary, and will depend on the law and the level of resulting harm.

The phrase 'duty of care' is used to explain the obligations that are implicit in your role as a nurse. You owe a duty of care to your patients, your colleagues, your employer, yourself and the public interest. A duty of care is not something that you can opt out of. It applies to all staff of all occupations and at all levels, to those working part time or full time, and to those in agency or temporary roles including students.

The people you care for are owed a duty of care from the moment they are accepted for treatment or a task is accepted and they receive services. All health and social care organisations have a duty of care, which provides a comprehensive service to citizens and demonstrates that, within the available resources, the appropriate priorities will be chosen.

There may be occasions when you or your employer cannot do everything that you consider needs to be done, but this does not mean the duty of care has been breached (UNISON, 2011). Resources are not limitless and as such the obligation of an employee and employer is to ensure that what is actually done is done safely and in an appropriate and timely manner (see the *NHS Constitution*; Department of Health, 2010). It should also be made clear what cannot be done.

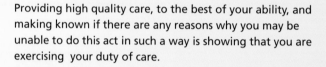

PEARLS OF WISDOM

Providing high quality care, to the best of your ability, and making known if there are any reasons why you may be unable to do this act in such a way is showing that you are exercising your duty of care.

You must follow a standard of reasonable care and you are expected to:

- keep your knowledge and skills up to date,
- provide a service of no less a quality than that to be expected based on the skills, responsibilities and range of activities within the profession,
- be in a position to know what must be done to ensure that the service is provided safely,
- keep accurate and contemporaneous records,
- not delegate work, or accept delegated work, unless it is clear that the person to whom the work is delegated is competent to carry out the work concerned in a safe and appropriately skilled manner,
- protect confidential information unless the wider duty of care or the public interest might justify disclosure.

As a practitioner you should not be asked and nor should you take on or perform any task that is beyond your level of competence. If you are asked to take on tasks that you are not properly equipped or trained to do you should decline and provide an explaination why.

As well as your duty of care you must also keep to the various standards of performance, conduct, competency and ethics outlined by the NMC in it code of professional conduct (Nursing and Midwifery Council, 2008). Every nurse registrant must read these standards and agree to keep to them, even if they are not practising. A breach of these standards carries the risk of suspension or removal from the professional register.

Student nurses and the duty of care

Student nurses also have a duty of care and therefore a legal liability with regards to the patient (Royal College of Nursing, 2011). However, the standard is different to that of a registered nurse. Students cannot be professionally accountable in the same way as fully trained practitioners. It is not expected that students will reach the standards of a registered nurse; they should be adequately prepared and supervised by an appropriately qualified member of staff. Throughout their education student nurses should aspire to meet the standards set by the NMC.

Should you be asked to undertake tasks which you consider you are not qualified to do then you must make that clear, in the first instance to your mentor or supervisor and if needed to your tutor or a more senior manager. Inappropriate delegation (whether by act or omission) is a very serious matter. Your mentor or supervisor and your university have a duty to ensure that you do not undertake tasks or responsibilities for which you are not qualified.

SECTION SUMMARY

All patients who use health services should be afforded a duty of care. When demonstrating their duty of care nurses must use reasonable care and skill. Patients are entitled to receive care of a standard that is considered to be appropriate to their condition. If the duty of care is breached, the patient may be able to cite a case for negligence.

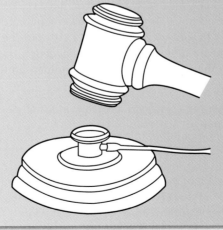

Negligence

Many cases of misconduct are associated with clinical negligence (sometimes called medical negligence). Negligence occurs when a nurse exposes a patient to a level of risk not common to the procedure being performed. All care interventions and procedures come with risks, but it can be deemed negligence in those cases when the level of risk exceeds what it would be if the procedure was performed by another nurse.

 I didn't know that when I chose to study nursing I also chose to study law. *Tanya, first year student nurse*

A registered nurse is deemed competent after completing a 3-year approved programme of study that meets the requirements laid down by the NMC (Nursing and Midwifery Council, 2010).

PEARLS OF WISDOM

Understanding how negligence is defined in nursing may help you appreciate the expected roles and standards, as well as what may be construed as negligence.

The basic and legal definition of negligence is breach of duty or injury. Standards of care in nursing usually mean those practices that a reasonably prudent nurse would use. So a good nurse (a nurse deemed competent) knows and understands ethics in the healthcare field and strives to provide an excellent standard of care to increase safety and to avoid negligence. However, mistakes do happen, and when they do they do not necessarily mean that negligence has occurred.

In England and Wales, for a person to succeed in a claim for negligence the claimant needs to prove that:

- the healthcare worker owed a duty to take care of the claimant and not cause injury,
- there was a breach of that duty to take care,
- breach of duty has caused harm to the claimant,
- damage or other losses have resulted from that harm.

The only outcome for a claimant that brings a successful clinical negligence claim is an award of damages. Courts cannot force a hospital or care provider to change its working practices or improve standards. It cannot discipline a health professional nor can it make a health professional apologise.

Duty of care

Previous sections of this chapter have already discussed a duty of care. Usually the complainant will have little difficulty in proving that the nurse, doctor or other healthcare worker (this will also apply to the student nurse) who are responsible for treating a patient owe a duty to take care of him or her.

It is essential to understand and reiterate once again that the law imposes a duty of care on practitioners, whether healthcare support workers, students, registered nurses, doctors or others, in those circumstances where it is 'reasonably foreseeable' that they might cause harm to patients through their actions or their failure to act (Cox, 2010).

The duty of care applies whether the task being undertaken involves feeding a patient or a complex surgical intervention. In both of these instances there is the chance for harm to occur. In this context, the question that arises concerns the standard of care that is expected of those practitioners performing these tasks. This is the legal liability the practitioner owes to the patient. By accepting the responsibility to perform a task the practitioner has to ensure that the task is performed competently, at least to the standard of the ordinarily competent practitioner in that type of task.

Nurses are absolved from their duty of care if a patient refuses care. However, the nurse must demonstrate that the patient was informed, acted in voluntarily manner (e.g. not coerced) and was competent to make that decision. As a result, even care that is life-saving in nature cannot be administered if the patient refuses. To do so would be to act against the principles of informed consent and that would constitute unlawful touching (Aveyard, 2004).

 ## Breach of duty

The complainant must be able to demonstrate that whatever the nurse did or did not do fell below the standard of a reasonably competent nurse in that particular field of nursing. The test of whether a nurse breached the duty of care owed to a patient is whether he or she has failed to meet the standard of a reasonable body of other practitioners also skilled in that field. This is known as the Bolam test (Bolam v Friern Hospital Management Committee [1957] 1 WLR 582). More recently, a court has stated that where a body of nursing or medical opinion is relied on to show that a particular nurse was not negligent it is also necessary to show that such opinion itself is logical and reasonable. What this means is that it is not enough that there is a body of opinion supporting the nurse; the body of opinion itself must be reasonable (Bolitho v City and Hackney Health Authority [1997] 3 WLR 1151).

The duty on the nurse to act in such a way that is reasonable applies whether the matter concerns treatment, diagnosis or advice given.

In some cases, and this can happen in the independent sector, a patient may have a contract with a nurse in respect of his or her treatment. In the absence of any specific provisions, the standard of care is the same as that described above. However, it should be noted that if a nurse guarantees a particular result then, if the nurse fails to produce that result, the nurse could be in breach of contract even if he or she has not in fact been negligent (think for example of those nurses who work independently in the aesthetic field).

Sometimes there is no other explanation except that there has been negligence. An example would be where a surgeon removed the wrong kidney. In these sorts of cases there is a presumption that the doctor was negligent and it is then up to him or her to prove otherwise.

 ## Causation

As well as proving that the nurse has failed to come up to the relevant standard of care, the claimant must also establish that this failure either directly caused the injuries alleged or significantly contributed to them. It is this aspect of the claim that is very often difficult to demonstrate; it may be easy to prove that the nurse did something wrong but it has to be shown that this failure caused the patient's injuries, which can be challenging. For example, a patient may be able to demonstrate that a consultant mental health nurse's diagnosis was wrong, but it is will be much harder to demonstrate that this has contributed to the person's present distress. There are some cases where there has been a very clear breach of duty, but there has been no damage as a result. In this scenario, no costs or compensation would be payable.

There may be occasions whereby the nurse caring for the person has admitted that there has been a breach of duty. However, this admission is not enough to determine that the person or employer is liable for any damages. For the person to establish liability it must be shown that the breach of duty has resulted in the damage.

 ## Burden of proof

The burden of proving negligence is on the claimant. The standard of proof is a 'balance of probabilities'; in other words, it is more likely than not that the defendant was negligent. The patient not the nurse has to prove that the nurse was negligent. The nurse (the defendant) does not have to prove that he or she was not negligent: the onus for this falls on the claimant (the patient).

 ## Avoiding allegations of negligence

Maintaining competence is essential if the nurse is to provide safe and high-quality care as well as ensuring that allegations of negligence are avoided. A competent nurse is well informed of contemporary practice and through continuing professional development (CPD) can demonstrate this if called to account (see Chapter 18). The competent nurse is diligent, demonstrates an awareness and an understanding of duties and works within professional and legal guidelines.

Examples of clinical negligence

There are many examples of clinical negligence and these can include negligence in relation to:

- provision of nursing care,
- surgery,
- medication,
- diagnosis,
- delay in treatment,
- psychiatric care,
- psychotherapy,
- counselling,
- dentistry,
- childbirth (including damage to the unborn child).

Negligence can also include things that have not been done but which should have been done; for example, not providing a person with the treatment they need, or failing to warn a person about the potential risks of a proposed treatment. Regardless of the kind of treatment, if all the elements set out above are present there is a potential claim for damages, but all the elements must be proven.

 ## Liability

Nurses and other healthcare professionals may be directly liable for their own negligent treatment. Their employers, often the NHS, the independent or voluntary care sectors, can be 'vicariously' liable for the negligence of their staff. As such, all nurses should have adequate indemnity insurance cover.

If the negligent nurse works for the NHS – for example, as a staff nurse – then it would be the health service employer that would be liable. The hospital pays the damages if a claim is successful. Nurses, doctors, students and other healthcare staff in the NHS are covered by the NHS. In the independent sector a clinic or private hospital will take out its own insurance. Nurses using the facilities of the clinic (for example, aesthetic nurses) will be independent contractors, and as such any claim should be against them as individual practitioners (the same applies for independent midwives). In almost all cases it will be the individual nurse who is sued. As stated, insurance is essential.

SECTION SUMMARY

There has been an increase over the years in the number of cases of clinical negligence. The NHS aims, and usually succeeds, in providing a safe and high level of care to the people who use its services. Negligence occurs when there is a breach of the legal duty of care owed to one person by another and the outcome results in damage being caused to that person. Clinical negligence is concerned with claims against nurses and other healthcare professionals and their employers. There are certain criteria that need to be satisfied to prove that clinical negligence has occurred.

 Consent

Consent to treatment is the principle that a person must give their permission before they receive any type of medical treatment. Consent is required from a patient irrespective of the treatment, from taking blood pressure to performing surgery. Most definitions of consent, according to Gillon (2003), are ambiguous. Basically, consent can mean to agree, accept or assent but, Wheeler (2012) warns, to simply agree or assent to something does not imply the notion of informed consent; in clinical practice there must be genuine agreement to consent.

The principle of consent is an important part of human rights law. For consent to be valid it has to be voluntary and informed and the person consenting must have the capacity to make the decision (see Table 16.2).

Table 16.2 Valid consent

Concept	Description
Voluntary	The decision to consent or not consent to treatment must be made alone and must not be due to pressure by nurses, medical staff, friends or family.
Informed	The person must be given full information about what the treatment includes, as well as the benefits and risks, whether there are reasonable alternative treatments and what may happen if treatment does not go ahead. Nurses and healthcare professionals should not withhold information just because it may upset or unnerve the person.
Capacity	The person must be capable of giving consent. This means that they understand the information given to them and they can use it to make an informed decision.

All adults are presumed to have the mental capacity to consent or refuse treatment, but there are some exceptions to this and they are if the person is:

- unable to take in or retain the information provided about their treatment or care,
- unable to understand the information that has been provided,
- unable to weigh up the information as part of the decision-making process.

The issue and assessment as to whether or not an adult lacks the capacity to consent is mainly down to the clinician who is providing the treatment or care, but nurses also have a responsibility to participate in discussions about the assessment of the person.

There are three over-riding professional responsibilities that nurses must give due regard to when obtaining consent:

1 to make the care of people their first concern and ensure they gain consent before they begin any form of treatment or care,
2 to ensure that the process of establishing consent is detailed, transparent and demonstrates a clear level of professional accountability,
3 to accurately record all discussions and decisions related to obtaining consent.

Valid consent must be given by a competent person (who may be a person lawfully appointed on behalf of the person) and it must be given voluntarily (there must be no coercion). Another person cannot give consent for an adult who has the capacity to consent. Exceptions to this are detailed in the next section.

Emergency situations

If an adult who becomes temporarily unable to consent due to, for example, being unconscious, they may be given treatment that is necessary to preserve life. When a case such as this arises the law permits treatment to be provided without the person's consent, as long as it is in the best interest of that person. The nurse must be sure that his or her actions are in the person's best interest.

Any medical intervention that is considered being in the person's best interest, but which can be delayed until they can consent, should be administered when the person is able to do so. There are exceptions to this; for example, where the person has issued an advanced directive that provides details of refusal of treatment.

Obtaining consent

Obtaining consent should be seen as a process as opposed to a one-off event. When the person is told about the proposed treatment and care, it is essential that the information be offered in a sensitive and understandable way. The nurse should give the person sufficient time to think about the information and also provide them with the opportunity to ask questions if they wish to. Nurses should never assume that the person they are caring for has sufficient knowledge for them to make a choice, even about basic treatment.

PEARLS OF WISDOM

You should never make assumptions about people because when we *assume* we can make an *ass* out of you and *me*:

ass u me

People should be involved in their care and the code of professional conduct (Nursing and Midwifery Council, 2008) supports involving people in the caregiving process, stating 'nurses must uphold the rights of people to be fully involved in decisions about their care'. One of the key issues associated with informed consent is the need to provide people with enough information that will enable them to decide whether or not to accept or decline the treatment and care offered. The nurse must respect and support the person's rights to either accept or decline any treatment and care that is being offered.

Failing to provide the person with sufficient information could lead to a complaint to the NMC or they may take legal action. Legal action is usually in the form of an allegation of negligence.

PEARLS OF WISDOM

You should provide people with information concerning their health in a way that they can understand it. You must be very careful when doing this so as not to patronise the person being cared for.

If consent has been obtained by deception or where insufficient information was given, this may result in an allegation of battery (in Scotland this is civil assault). It is only in the most extreme of cases that the criminal law is likely to be involved.

Who obtains consent?

The nurse who is proposing to perform a procedure should obtain consent, but there may be some situations where this can be delegated to another. When choosing to delegate the nurse should:

- ascertain that the person being delegated to is able to carry out the instructions given,
- check that the outcome of the delegated task conforms to the required standards.

Normally it is the person performing the procedure who should be the person obtaining consent. There may be some circumstances, when the nurse may seek consent on behalf of another colleague if the nurse has been specially trained for that particular area of practice.

On some occasions nurses, although caring for the person, are not responsible for either obtaining consent or for performing the procedure. In these instances the nurse is often best placed to know and to judge what information the person needs in order to make a decision.

Nurses should be aware of the importance of communication within the team and should raise any concerns regarding a person's understanding of a procedure. This should be communicated appropriately. Difficulties in understanding might be as a result of language differences. Interpreters can sometimes help to assist in such cases. The NMC code of professional conduct (Nursing and Midwifery Council, 2008) states that nurses must keep colleagues informed when they are sharing the care of others; they must also make sure that they make arrangements to meet people's language and communication needs; this could involve ensuring the availability of an interpreter.

Types of consent

There are many ways the person in your care can demonstrate their consent. If the person agrees to treatment and care they can do this verbally; they can also do it in writing or by implying (when they are cooperating) that they are agreeing. It is important to remember that they may also withdraw or refuse their consent in the same way. Verbal consent, or consenting by implication, will be sufficient evidence in the majority of cases. When the care intervention is deemed risky, lengthy or complex then written consent should be obtained. Written consent stands as a record that discussions have occurred and the person has been involved. The person may refuse treatment and if this is the case it is important that a written record of this is made. The nurse should record the discussions and decisions.

ACTIVITY 16.3

Think about your work in the clinical setting and take some time to reflect about the various ways in which consent has been obtained when you or others work with people you care for.

Remember the various ways in which consent can be given:
- verbally,
- nonverbally; for example, when the person raises their arm to indicate he or she is happy for you to take a blood pressure,
- in writing, by signing a consent form.

If a person refuses consent

In law a competent adult can give or refuse their consent to treatment, even if that refusal could result in harm or death (Wheeler, 2012). The nurse has a duty to respect their refusal in the same way that they would respect their consent. It is essential that the person is fully informed and, when necessary, other members of the healthcare team are involved. Refusal to consent, as with consent itself, must be recorded.

Advanced directives or living wills are recognised in law and by the NMC. These documents are made in advance of a particular condition arising and express the person's treatment choices, including decisions not to accept further treatment in particular circumstances.

Although they may not necessarily be legally binding, they can provide very useful information about the wishes of a person who has become unable to make a decision.

 ## Those under 16 years

If the person is a minor (under 16 years of age) then the nurse must be aware of any local protocols and legislation that may affect their care or treatment. Consent of people under 16 is very complex, and it is suggested that local, legal or professional organisation's advice be sought. Those under the age of 16 are usually considered to lack the capacity to consent or to refuse treatment. The parents, or those with parental responsibility, retain the right to consent or refuse unless the child is judged to have significant understanding and intelligence to make up his or her own mind about it.

People who are aged 16 or 17 years are thought to be able to consent for themselves, although it is considered good practice to involve the parents. Parents or those with parental responsibility can override the refusal of a child of any age up to 18 years. It may be necessary to seek an order from the court in exceptional circumstances. It is unusual for child minders, teachers and other adults caring for the child to give consent.

In Scotland the Age of Legal Capacity (Scotland) Act 1991 provides the current position on the legal capacity of children, including giving or withholding consent to treatment. The law is generally similar to that in England and Wales. There is one important difference, however, which is that a parent's consent cannot override a refusal of consent by a competent child. In Scotland a child under the age of 16 has the legal capacity to consent to his or her own treatment where, according to the Act, 'in the opinion of the qualified medical practitioner attending to him/her, he/she is capable of understanding the nature and possible consequences of the procedure or treatment'.

 ## Mental capacity

When a person is judged or considered incapable of providing consent, or where the wishes of a mentally incapacitated person appear to be different to the interests of that person, the nurse caring for that particular person should be involved in assessing their care or treatment. It is important that nurses are aware of the legislation concerning mental capacity, ensuring that people who lack capacity remain central to the decision-making process and are fully safeguarded (Nursing and Midwifery Council, 2008).

There are certain circumstances that the courts have identified when referral should be made to them for a ruling on lawfulness prior to a procedure being undertaken. These are:

- 🜍 sterilisation for contraceptive purposes,
- 🜍 donation of regenerative tissue such as bone marrow,
- 🜍 withdrawal of nutrition and hydration from a patient in a persistent vegetative state,
- 🜍 where there is doubt as to the person's capacity or best interests.

Other legal acts allow people who are over the age of 16 to appoint a proxy decision maker. This person has the legal power to give consent to medical treatment when the patient loses the capacity to consent. The various acts require medical practitioners to take into account, so far as is reasonable and practicable, the views of the patient's nearest relative and their carer.

Mental health acts

For those people who are detained under the applicable mental health legislation, the principles of consent continue to apply for conditions that are not related to the mental disorder. Nurses involved in the care or treatment of people detained under the relevant mental health legislation have to ensure that they are aware of the circumstances and safeguards required for providing treatment and care without consent.

 I was allocated to an acute mental health ward. The issues of consent, human rights, liberty and freedom of choice really brought home to me the importance of ensuring that the person must be at the heart of all we do. I used to take all of those things for granted and I never gave them a second thought. Not anymore. *Simon, second year student*

Mental Capacity Act 2005

This Act seeks to empower people who lack 'capacity', helping to ensure that they remain at the centre of the decision-making process and to safeguard them and those who work with them. The Act makes clear who can take decisions, in which situations and how they should do this. It also allows people to plan ahead for a time when they may lose capacity. The Act became fully effective in April 2007 and applies to England and Wales, providing a statutory framework to empower and protect vulnerable people who are unable to make their own decisions. It applies to those aged 16. Scotland has similar legislation in place with The Adults with Incapacity (Scotland) Act 2000. The Mental Health (Northern Ireland) Order 1986 covers capacity.

There are five key principles underpinning the Act.

1 A presumption of capacity: adults have the right to make their own decisions and must be assumed to have capacity to do so unless proved otherwise.
2 The right for individuals to be supported to make their own decisions and to be given all appropriate help before anyone infers that they cannot make their own decisions.
3 Individuals must retain the right to make what might be seen as eccentric or unwise decisions.
4 Anything done for or on behalf of people without capacity must be in their best interests.
5 Anything done for or on behalf of people without capacity should be the least restrictive of their basic rights and freedoms.

Summary

There are many key links between the law and the code of professional conduct (Nursing and Midwifery Council, 2008), and nursing and its many forms are inherently linked with the law and ethics. Understanding the ethical and legal aspects associated with care provision can help you practice in a safe and professional manner. Nursing protocols and procedures are intended to help nurses respond to clinical situations in a safe and appropriate way. They provide the framework for the management of a specific disorder or clinical situation. Failing to adhere to protocol and policy can result in legal action being taken as well as being called to account by the NMC for any actions and omissions.

Nurses owe a duty of care to the people in their care. When a nurse acts in a careless way and this action results in harm or injury the nurse will be liable for negligence. There are certain conditions that must be established by the claimant (the patient) to establish negligence.

In clinical practice consent is more than merely agreeing, accepting or assenting to something, it is complex and has at the heart of it patient autonomy: acting in the person's best interests. The Human Rights Act 1998 determines that people have a right to consent to their body being touched prior to care provision. Equally as important is that they also have right to refuse care. There are several exceptions to this right and these are also complex: the nurse is advised to seek expert opinion. Consent can come in many forms; for example, verbally, nonverbally and in written form.

References

Aveyard, H. (2004) The patient who refuses nursing care. *Journal of Medical Ethics* 30, 346–50
Collins, S. and Patel, S. (2009) Development of clinical policies and guidelines in acute settings. *Nursing Standard* 23(27), 42–7
Cox, C. (2010) Legal responsibility and accountability. *Nursing Management* 17(3), 18–20
Department of Health (2010) *The NHS Constitution*. Department of Health, London

Friedman, J.W. (2007) Musings on policy. Director's memo. *Policy and Practice* 65(3), 3

Gillon, R. (2003) *Philosophical Medical Ethics*. Wiley, Chichester

Nursing and Midwifery Council (2008) The Code: Standards of Conduct, Performance and Ethics for Nurses and Midwives. Nursing and Midwifery Council, London

Nursing and Midwifery Council (2010) *Standards for Pre Registration Nursing Education*. http://standards.nmc-uk.org/PublishedDocuments/Standards%20for%20pre-registration%20nursing%20education%2016082010.pdf

Open Clinical (2011) *Clinical Pathways: Multi-disciplinary Plans of Best Clinical Practice*. www.openclinical.org/clinicalpathways.html

Royal College of Nursing (2011) *Accountability and Delegation: What You Need to Know*. Royal College of Nursing, London

Sudduth, A.L. (2008) Program evaluation. In Milstead, J.A. (ed.), *Health Policy and Politics: A Nurse's Guide*. Jones and Bartlett, Sudbury, pp. 171–96

UNISON (2011) *UNISON Duty of Care Handbook. For Members Working in Health and Social Care*. UNISON, London

Wheeler, H. (2012) *Law, Ethics and Professional Issues for Nursing. A Reflective and Portfolio-Building Approach*. Routledge, London

Working in Partnership Programme (2006) *Using Protocols, Standards, Policies and Guidelines to Enhance Confidence and Career Development, General Practice Nurse Toolkit*. www.wipp.nhs.uk/tools_gpn/toolu5_using_protocols.php

 ## Resources

Mind

www.mind.org.uk/help/rights_and_legislation

A good resource, providing information about a variety of legal issues from a mental health perspective.

Royal College of Nursing

www.rcn.org.uk/support/legal

The RCN is the largest professional union for nursing in the UK, with around 400 000 members in the NHS and the private and independent sectors. The RCN has a number of legal resources available.

UNISON

www.unison.org.uk

UNISON is the UK's largest public service union, representing more than 1.3 million people who provide vital services to the public. UNISON has a number of legal resources available.

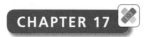

CHAPTER 17

Clinical Academic Careers

You are fully aware that nursing is a very popular and rewarding career with a number of diverse opportunities and that career-development prospects are good. Nurses work in a variety of settings, such as hospitals, doctors' surgeries, universities, people's homes, schools and industry. When registered as a nurse you may want to work on the front line, working in accident and emergency, or you might want to work in a local care home or have a job with more of a community-based focus. Regardless of your choice you will be making a difference.

In contemporary society there are a number of high public expectations and nurses need to respond to these to reinforce public confidence in the profession and to ensure that the care provided is of a high quality. Coming through 3 years of undergraduate nurse education and securing your name on the professional register is something to be very proud of. You have demonstrated your ability to move from being a novice nurse to a competent practitioner: the next stage of your career begins now. In Benner's terms (Benner 1984) the next stages are to become proficient and then to become an expert practitioner.

Nurses are already playing a key part in research, practice and education in the NHS and social care. Nurses lead and contribute to the generation of new knowledge about care and treatment, supporting the development of a dynamic and innovative world-class workforce that actively seeks out the best evidence to help improve outcomes and experiences for people.

The Student Nurse Toolkit: An Essential Guide for Surviving Your Course, First Edition. Ian Peate.
© 2013 John Wiley & Sons, Ltd. Published 2013 by John Wiley & Sons, Ltd.

Transferrable skills

All of the skills you have developed and honed throughout your nurse education are transferable skills. This fact will enable you to adapt these skills to the various situations that you encounter as you progress through your nursing career. The career opportunities available for nurses are continuing to grow: doors are opening where hitherto they had been firmly shut.

The Department of Health has placed much emphasis on transferable skills and this can be identified when the Knowledge and Skills Framework (or KSF) (Department of Health, 2004) is considered. The Knowledge and Skills Framework is used by all staff in the NHS (except doctors and dentists) to consider the comparable skills in a number of posts.

ACTIVITY 17.1

Take the job description of a band 5 staff nurse and look at the Knowledge and Skills Framework indicators. Now match these with your current skills and attributes and this will give you some idea how much more development you will need before you become registered. As a first year student you will still have some way to go but, as a nearly qualified third year student, your skill set should be close to that required of a band 5 staff nurse.

As part of your pre-registration education the curriculum offers a flexible principle-based approach that is built around patient pathways, with a strong academic foundation and interdisciplinary learning. The programme you studied or are still studying provides you with transferable skills. This is in contrast to the older-style system that resembled a one-size-fits-all approach, which often struggled to balance academic and practical learning and was reflective of healthcare yesterday and not tomorrow.

A report from the four Chief Nursing Officers of the UK, *Modernising Nursing Careers: Setting the Direction* (Department of Health, 2006), mapped out the future shape of nursing in response to a variety of Government priorities in health and social care policy. As has been demonstrated in previous chapters of this book, healthcare is moving away from a secondary care-focused arena to one in which primary and community care are central. Much more emphasis is being placed on public health and preventive medicine in a health service that is striving to maintain health and well-being as opposed to focusing on individual sickness events. As part of this there is greater emphasis being made on chronic health conditions and self-care. Healthcare is also aiming to be more responsive to patient needs and expectations, with patients at the centre. People are now expected to take a greater role in their own health management and so people will require more access to information and a more active participation in healthcare. Nurses and other healthcare professionals must involve families and lay carers when they provide care. There is also a need to provide greater choice for patients with more care being available closer to and within the home.

The flexibility of the undergraduate nursing curriculum is fundamental in giving nurses a foundation for the development of diverse careers. This approach also allows movement between roles, both within and outside the NHS. In so doing it goes some way to meeting the Chief Nursing Officers' aspirations.

PEARLS OF WISDOM

Discuss your future nursing career with your personal tutor, who may be able to suggest career trajectories that have not yet occurred to you.

Your undergraduate pre-registration nursing programme has laid down the foundation for whatever pathway you choose in nursing, including a clinical academic career. Clinical academic careers are relatively new in the nursing profession and are now gathering momentum. This option will not suit all graduates but it is one that you should consider.

SECTION SUMMARY

A professional qualification is essential for jobs within nursing. Undertaking a programme of study like nursing provides you with a range of professional and technical skills, including the ability to function effectively as part of a multidisciplinary team and to support and advise patients and their families. You also develop the ability to assess, analyse, monitor and evaluate the care you deliver. Undergraduate nursing programmes of study can provide you with additional transferable skills and personal qualities including flexibility, organisation and time management, leadership and the ability to conduct research. Your programme provides you with the opportunity to develop problem-solving and decision-making skills, equipping you with confidence and the ability to deal with a diverse and changing profession.

Modern nursing careers

Nursing careers yesterday, today and tomorrow have been and will be in a constant state of flux; this is given in the light of the discussion earlier in this chapter concerning the changing health and social care landscape. Regardless of where a nurse works there are five key elements associated with their role and function:

1 practice,
2 education,
3 training and development,
4 quality and service development,
5 leadership, management and supervision.

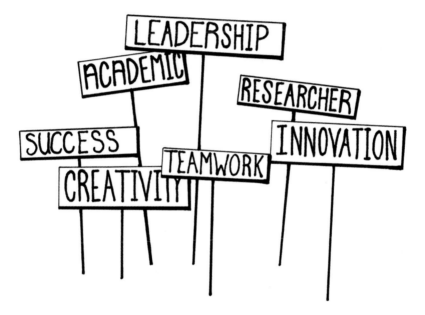

The nursing workforce will still be required to:

- organise care around the needs of people,
- ensure that people have a good experience of nursing based on safe, effective, high-quality care,
- work in a variety of settings, traversing hospital and community care, making more use of technologies such as telemedicine,
- have the skills and competencies to care for older people and people with long-term conditions, as well as people who may have both physical and mental health needs,
- be able to develop, use and evaluate preventative and health promotion interventions,

- work for different employers, taking opportunities for self-employment and entrepreneurship where appropriate,
- be made up of sufficient numbers of nurses who have advanced level skills to meet demand,
- work as leaders and members of multidisciplinary teams inside and across health and social care sectors,
- work with new types of practitioners; for example, assistant practitioners,
- deliver high productivity and best value for money.

Over the years nurses have been taking on and developing new roles and responsibilities, contributing significantly to improvements in patient care. Nurses have been instrumental in reducing waiting times, improving the quality of care and making services more accessible. New senior clinical roles, such as clinical nurse specialists, nurse consultants and modern matrons and community matrons, have been introduced and developed in England. These ensure that experienced and highly skilled nurses stay close to patient care. In Scotland there has been a review of the role of the senior charge nurse, which will help to create modern charge nurse roles to enable frontline clinical leaders to make the most out of their contribution to delivering safe and effective care.

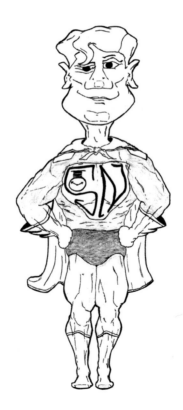

A career structure is needed that will enable nurses to work in diverse care settings as well as taking on changing roles and responsibilities, pursuing education when they need it and developing a varied mix of generalist and specialist skills as required. A modern nursing career structure is required, and Table 17.1 considers how the traditional career structure compares to this new career structure.

Table 17.1 Traditional career structure compared to a proposed new career structure

Traditional	...to...	Proposed
Old-fashioned image of nursing and nursing careers dictated by media stereotypes		An up-to-date picture of nursing careers characterised by opportunity and diversity
A nursing workforce with a focus on hospital care		Care taking place both inside and outside hospital with nurses moving between More nurses starting their career in community-based settings
A single entry point to nursing		A career framework that permits nursing to 'grow its own' with several entry points for those taking up nursing as a second career or as mature entrants
Working for the NHS as a single employer		Variety of provision providing different employers and employment models including NHS Foundation Trusts, self-employment and social enterprises
An education system with a one-size-fits-all approach, struggling to balance academic and practical learning and reflective of healthcare today not tomorrow		A flexible principle-based curriculum that is built around patient pathways, with a strong academic foundation and interdisciplinary learning
Careers characterised by increasing specialisation or promotion out of practice with consequences for those who want to step off or change trajectory		A framework that supports movement between career pathways, practice, management and education, valuing and rewarding different career types
Increasing specialisation and sub-specialisation		Better balance of generalists and specialists to provide integrated networks of urgent, specialist and continuing care

Table 17.1 *(continued)*

Traditional	...to...	Proposed
Careers defined by specialty or setting		Careers built around patient pathways using competence as the means for greater movement and flexibility
Organisation-based careers with an excess of titles		Patient pathway-based careers focusing on nursing roles rather than titles
Role determined by title		Nursing roles defined according to patient need: providing intervention that is timely, accurate and swift
Nursing teams hierarchically managed		Nursing teams more self-directed and professionally accountable
Nurses involved predominantly in care provision		Nurses leading, coordinating and commissioning care, as well as giving care, to bring about change measured by health gain and health outcomes
Care dictated by custom and practice, tradition and ritual		Care that is evidence-based with critical thinking, assisted by new technology

Source: adapted Department of Health (2006).

With emphasis on more modern nursing career structures, this will promote greater movement, flexibility and diversity than ever before. Nursing staff will be able to move between clinical, management and academic careers and also into different organisations and sectors. There is a commitment to enable nurses (and other health and social care staff) to move between health and social services, independent and voluntary sectors, or increasingly into social services, housing and schools. As people are being provided with more services in or closer to home, there will be many opportunities for those nurses in acute settings to follow patients and work wholly or partially outside hospital.

> I have just finished working in a drug and alcohol rehabilitation unit and this is definitely what I want to specialise in. I am going to apply for a job with social services as a nurse working only with social workers. I will be the only nurse in the team.
> *Jade, third year student nurse*

There is a need to develop careers in education and research taking place in or between service and the university. Leadership roles have taken nurses into directorships and chief executive posts, into government, professional or employee organisations as well as regulation. All types of careers can lead to entrepreneurship through social enterprise, self-employment, franchised services or small business operations.

New career structures will encourage movement and progression as well as providing rich opportunities for nurses who want to stay where they are and work as locally as possible. They can also support more personalised career paths, meeting the needs and aspirations of individuals at different stages of life.

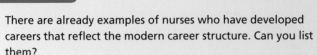

ACTIVITY 17.2

There are already examples of nurses who have developed careers that reflect the modern career structure. Can you list them?

The Commission for the Future of Nursing (2010), in its report *Front Line Care*, recommended an urgent review of the integration of practice, education and research, to facilitate sustainable clinical academic careers and further develop research skills. The Government responded to the report by supporting the integration and outlined the responsibility of the NHS, providers and universities to develop flexible career pathways and gave explicit support for research training pathways. The modernisation of career structures across other types healthcare professions is currently being addressed. Nursing is not the only profession; scientific careers, allied health professionals and medicine are also in the process of being modernised.

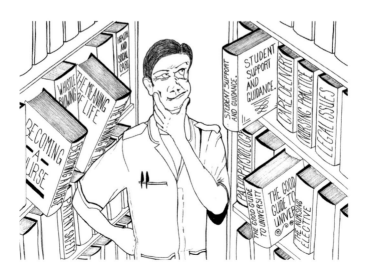

SECTION SUMMARY

Modernising nursing careers has the aim of developing a competent and flexible nursing workforce, updating career pathways and choices for nurses. The new career framework will prepare nurses to lead in a healthcare system that is constantly changing. Modern nursing careers are important, not only to meet public and patient needs, expectations and views but also in terms of the viability of the future nursing workforce as recognised key leaders and deliverers of healthcare in the future. The aims are also important in terms of future nursing recruitment and ensuring that nursing is seen as an attractive career option.

Clinical academic careers

The role of a clinical academic nurse is one of the responses to the Chief Nursing Officers' desires to modernise nursing careers (Department of Health, 2006). A clinical academic nurse combines and integrates clinical and academic work, as opposed to having to pursue one role at the expense of the other. Academic duties associated with the role may include research, teaching or both. A clinical academic career fosters clinical excellence, research and teaching in a systemic relationship. It has the potential to offer flexible career opportunities that can sustain and develop clinical skills as well as offering opportunities to become proficient researchers and educators (UK Clinical Research Collaboration, 2007).

Clinical academic posts are usually joint appointments between a healthcare provider and higher education institution. It is often the case that one organisation will hold the substantive contract of employment of the clinical nurse academic, establishing honorary contracts with the intention of facilitating working across organisational boundaries.

Clinical academics are making a demonstrable impact on the quality of care and the productivity of services. They contribute to the generation of new knowledge about care and treatment and actively seek out the best evidence to help them improve outcomes and experiences for people. The Department of Health (2012) has outlined its aspirations to support the growth of the nursing, midwifery and allied health professions' clinical academic workforce and to embed and sustain these roles (see Box 17.1).

Scotland has also produced national guidance to support the development of Nursing, Midwifery and Allied Health Professions clinical academic research careers; there are similarities with both approaches in Scotland and England. This

Box 17.1 Clinical academic careers

Work in a range of clinical academic environments

Nurses do not just work in hospitals. Clinical academic careers can take nurses into a range of clinical and academic environments; for example, people's homes, nursing homes, community clinics and schools. More and more nurses will deliver and lead care in many different contexts including acute and critical care, first contact, access and urgent care, family and public health, mental health and long-term care.

Pursue an integrated clinical and academic career

Those nurses who chose a clinical academic career pathway will pursue a single integrated career combining clinical practice and research or clinical practice and education, as opposed to having to choose a career in one or the other. These nurses will exercise their clinical and research/education responsibilities concurrently. The role will be clinically relevant and practice-focused.

Learn, train and develop

To progress personally and professionally from one level to another there are requirements in terms of qualifications and training. Nurses thinking about this pathway will need to actively evaluate and plan their professional development to ensure incremental steps to develop knowledge and intellectual abilities, personal qualities and self-management skills. Pursuing the necessary education and training will equip the clinical academic nurse to ensure the people they care for experience high-quality, safe and effective care and that they excel in their chosen research or education pathway.

Move up and around

Once registered as a nurse, nurses will have reached level 5 as a healthcare practitioner on the NHS Career Framework, undergoing a period of preceptorship. As the nurse progresses they will continue to build their skills as a practitioner, partner and leader. As a clinical academic the nurse opts to build knowledge and skills in practice and research and/or education, gradually developing clinical expertise and specialising in a particular area of practice.

Source: adapted Department of Health (2012).

approach includes a Clinical Academic Research Career (CARC) Framework with accompanying principles (NHS Education for Scotland, 2011). The key aims are to provide a sustainable and consistent structure to guide clinical research collaborations and role development for the benefit of those people who use services and quality improvements in research in the university sector and NHS Scotland.

 ## The benefits of clinical academic roles

Clinical academic roles allow nurses to bring together roles, and integrate knowledge, skills and experience, in clinical practice and research (although these roles could be education-focused as opposed to research-based). The clinical academic nurse uses knowledge and experience of clinical practice to inform the research process and uses research and evidence to enhance the quality and efficacy of clinical practice. In this instance research is focused on finding solutions to problems that matter most to patients, their families and service providers and clinical practice is informed by evidence about what works and is best for patients and their families.

Clinical academic roles can provide opportunities for nurses to develop and advance their knowledge and skills in research and clinical practice at the same time and to amalgamate these to improve both their and others' research and practice. Finch (2009) notes that change cannot be immediate and that it will need to go on being positively supported with additional funds used strategically, building up both capability and capacity.

ACTIVITY 17.3

What are some of the challenges or barriers to advancing the modernising nursing careers agenda? How might they be addressed or overcome?

 ## Clinical academic role descriptors

There are a number of ways in which a nurse can pursue a clinical academic career, and indeed there may be opportunities to begin to develop learning and experiences relevant to this career pathway as a pre-registration undergraduate student. Following initial registration, a nurse can engage in a clinical academic pathway, gaining early clinical experience in a research-rich clinical practice environment, maintaining his or her links with research and/or maintaining clinical practice while working in a research role.

The UK Clinical Research Collaboration (2007) recommendations on clinical academic careers set out to determine a clearly identified and properly resourced career track for a proportion of nurses who wish to pursue a clinical academic career and who are likely to lead future programmes of clinical and health-related research. It must be clearly acknowledged that not all nurses can or want to pursue a clinical academic career.

Latter *et al.* (2009) have set out a model clinical academic career framework for nurses, midwives and allied health professionals who wish to combine clinical and academic roles. Clinical academic pathways can be divided into a variety of levels, beginning at level 5 and with the potential of developing to the highest level, level 9.

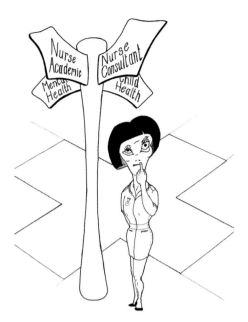

 ## Summary

The key aim of clinical academic careers is to combine research and education with a clinical career to improve the translation of research into clinical practice. A clinical academic nurse is a nurse who is engaged in both clinical and academic duties. The academic duties can include research, teaching or both. Such a career for nurses brings together clinical excellence, research and teaching in a systemic relationship. It should offer flexible career opportunities that sustain and develop clinical skills and offer opportunities to become proficient researchers and educators.

Undergraduate pre-registration nursing programmes have laid the foundation for whatever pathway the nurse chooses in his or her nursing career; one pathway is a clinic academic career. Clinical academic careers are fairly new in the nursing profession and are now gaining momentum. It is acknowledged that this option will not suit all graduates but it is one that you might want to consider.

 ## References

Benner, P. (1984) *From Novice to Expert. Excellence and Power in Clinical Nursing Practice.* Addison-Wesley, Menlo Park, CA

Commission for the Future of Nursing (2010) *Front Line Care.* http://webarchive .nationalarchives.gov.uk/20100331110400/http://cnm.independent.gov.uk/wp-content/ uploads/2010/03/front_line_care.pdf

Department of Health (2004) *The NHS Knowledge and Skills Framework (NHS KSF) and the Development Review Process (October 2004).* Department of Health, London

Department of Health (2006) *Modernising Nursing Careers: Setting the Direction*. Department of Health, London

Department of Health (2012) *A Strategy for Developing Clinical Academic Researchers within Nursing, Midwifery and the Allied Health Professions*. Department of Health, London

Finch, J. (2009) The importance of clinical academic careers in nursing. *Journal of Research in Nursing* 14(2), 103–5

Latter, S., Macleod Clark, J., Geddes, C. and Kitsell, F. (2009) Implementing a clinical academic career pathway in nursing; criteria for success and challenges ahead. *Journal of Research in Nursing* 14(2), 137–48

NHS Education for Scotland (2011) *National Guidance for Clinical Academic Research Careers for Nursing, Midwifery and Allied Health Professions in Scotland*. www.nes.scot.nhs.uk/media/241642/nmahp_national_guidance_for_clinical_academic_research_careers__mar_20

UK Clinical Research Collaboration (2007) *Developing the Best Research Professionals. Report of the UKCRC Sub-Committee for Nurses in Clinical Research (Workforce)*. UK Clinical Research Collaboration, London

 ## Resources

Department of Health
www.dh.gov.uk
This website gives you access to the full modernising health careers archives and updates.

NHS Career Planner for Nurses
http://nursingcareers.nhsemployers.org
The Nursing Career Framework is an interactive tool designed to help you plan and explore your future steps in nursing. It will help you to map out your desired career pathway.

NHS Scotland
www.show.scot.nhs.uk
Information is available on this site that can provide you with insight into clinical academic careers.

CHAPTER 18

Preceptorship and Continuing Professional Development

WHAT THIS CHAPTER CONTAINS

- Transitions and expectations
- Preceptorship
- Preceptorship framework
- An overview of continuing professional development and the NMC standards

Your education as a student nurse will no doubt have been rewarding. It may have also been physically, mentally and emotionally challenging. You have made it, so what is next for you? Well, the journey is only just beginning, and so is the learning.

The final year as a student will have felt very different to the previous 2 years. As the time came for you to graduate and register with the NMC you may have been apprehensive and anxious about people's (and your own) expectations of you. During the last year of your studies you would have been given more responsibility and more autonomy, and you would have been looked up to by the junior students with whom you worked. In that final year others would have been expecting more from you, that you would be working at a higher level from an academic and practical perspective. Your learning would have been more independent, no longer requiring so much guidance from others. In the practice setting you would also have been expected to be more of a team worker, a team leader and a decision maker, bringing together and putting into action all the knowledge and skills you have mastered over the previous years.

The Student Nurse Toolkit: An Essential Guide for Surviving Your Course, First Edition. Ian Peate.
© 2013 John Wiley & Sons, Ltd. Published 2013 by John Wiley & Sons, Ltd.

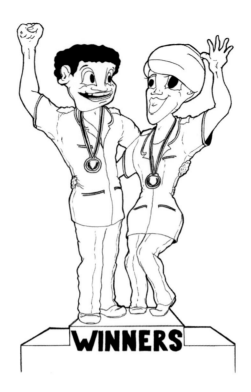

 ## Transitions and expectations

Kramer (1974) coined the term 'reality shock' in reference to the transition from student to qualified nurse. This transition period can be a difficult one, associated with a steep learning curve.

You might be terrified about leaving the protected world of the university and being a student, but the badge that used to say student nurse now says staff nurse. Try not to worry. During your time as a student you have had a variety of experiences and you have been exposed to many theoretical and practical aspects in educational and practice settings. Even as a student nurse you had to make your own decisions and you contributed a great deal to the health and well-being of many people, although granted you always had someone to look to for advice and insight. Many students (not just you) cite leaving behind the world of being a student as one of their greatest fears.

The people you work with in your first post as a staff nurse will not expect to see an expert arrive for duty on the first day. You will be allocated a mentor and/or a preceptor and there will be many other people around you from whom you can learn.

> *Just when I thought it was all over. Learn as much as you can but also know that the learning does not stop when you qualify, it goes on and on. Jamelia, third year student*

The public and the profession expect that when a nurse becomes qualified they are able to demonstrate a high level of knowledge, understanding and application of high-order skills, with both the people they care for as well as other members of the multidisciplinary team. These expectations should not come as a surprise to you; they are the skills that you have been developing on your journey to qualifying as a registered nurse. They are the requirements the NMC has of you through its standards of competence (Nursing and Midwifery Council, 2010). The five essential skills clusters (see Chapter 6) are:

- care, compassion and communication,
- organisational aspects of care,
- infection prevention and control,
- attending to and meeting needs such as nutrition and fluid management,
- medicines management.

When you register with the NMC there comes with this privilege a change in professional accountability, together with wider clinical, management, research and teaching responsibilities. Expectations and dynamics associated with your professional relationships change when you become a registered nurse. People will expect you to know the answer, be they students, doctors, patients or their families. You will certainly experience a number of challenging situations as you take the lead in care delivery.

Your assessments as a student nurse will demonstrate to the NMC that you are competent in the areas of:

- professional values,
- communication skills,
- decision making,
- leadership,
- personal and professional development.

You will be scrutinised and supported by others as you perform your work and this is only right, as the safety of the people you care for is paramount. Providing support for newly qualified health professionals through preceptorship has been advocated as one way of enhancing patient care. It helps new practitioners to develop their clinical skills and encourages workforce retention by supporting new nurses in their transition from student to registered practitioner (National Nursing Research Unit, 2009).

Write a list of all the modules you have completed on your nursing programme so far. If you are at the end of your programme of study this will be a long list. The idea is that by looking at this list (newer students can add to it as they progress on their programme) you should be feeling a little more confident in your actual and perceived competence. Your programme of study has equipped you to be a safe, competent practitioner.

Preparation for the transition from student to qualified nurse is often incorporated into the final year teaching modules (Broad *et al.*, 2011). This is most successful when a partnership approach is adopted; for example, when university and trust colleagues deliver the content.

SECTION SUMMARY

Moving from student nurse to qualified nurse is the result of 3 years' study and you can be congratulated on this achievement: you should be proud to be a registered nurse.
It can also bring with it with some tensions and anxiety. People will be expecting different things from you now that your badge says staff nurse; you will also be expecting different things from youself.

You have been deemed competent by the NMC, and you have the knowledge, skills and attitude to make a difference to the lives of people in your care. It has been acknowledged that newly qualified staff nurses need some assistance in adapting to the role of staff nurse and to make the transition from student to registered nurse. This help is available in the form of preceptorship.

> I know I know my stuff; I just need to do it now.
> *Rob, third year student nurse*

 ## Preceptorship

It has been accepted that nurses should be provided with some form of preceptorship and supervision in their new role for a period of time once they have completed their programme of study. This allows them time to settle into the new role. One of the key aims of preceptorship is to give nurses the best possible start because what happens to nurses at the beginning of their careers is crucial. Through preceptorship the aim is to nurture and develop newly qualified nurses to develop lifelong careers in nursing.

It has been recognised that the time following registration as a nurse can be a challenging, and good support and guidance during this period is essential. Newly registered nurses who are able to manage the transition successfully provide effective care more quickly; they will feel better about their role and they are more likely to remain within the profession (Department of Health, 2010). This means they will make a greater contribution to patient care, ensuring that the benefits from the investment in their education are maximised.

ACTIVITY 18.2

Before you move on, put together your own definition of preceptorship. Think about what you might need and what you would like as you make the transition from a student nurse to a registered nurse.

What is preceptorship?

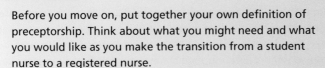

There are a number of definitions of preceptorship to choose from. The National Nursing Research Unit (2009) notes that there is some confusion surrounding the concept of preceptorship (particularly in the North American literature) in that it is used to refer to support for student nurses as well as support for newly qualified nurses. In 2006 the NMC defined preceptorship as:

> A period [of preceptorship] to guide and support all newly qualified practitioners to make the transition from student to develop their practice further. (Nursing and Midwifery Council, 2006)

A High Quality Workforce: NHS Next Stage Review (Department of Health, 2008) describes preceptorship as:

> A foundation period [of preceptorship] for practitioners at the start of their careers which will help them begin the journey from novice to expert.

The Department of Health (2010) uses the following definition of preceptorship:

> A period of structured transition for the newly registered practitioner during which he or she will be supported by a preceptor, to develop their confidence as an autonomous professional, refine skills, values and behaviours and to continue on their journey of life-long learning.

ACTIVITY 18.3

Consider again all three definitions above and then go back to your definition, the one you wrote for Activity 18.2. Of the three definitions provided here, which one is closest to yours?

The term preceptor can also be a problem to define. It can refer to a registered practitioner who has been given a formal responsibility to support a newly registered practitioner through preceptorship. A newly registered practitioner can be defined as a nurse who is entering employment for the first time after registration with the NMC. This can include those who are recently graduated students, those returning to practice, those entering a new part of the register (for example, community public health specialists) and overseas-prepared practitioners who have complied with the requirements of, and are registered with, the NMC. While engaged in preceptorship newly registered nurses may be referred to as a 'preceptee'.

Just as it is important to understand what preceptorship is, it is also important to know what it is not. You will have to have a clear understanding of the limits of preceptorship if you are to get the most out of it. Preceptors and preceptees must be aware that there are other processes and systems used in the workplace to manage performance and ability with respect to the competency of the newly registered staff nurse. Preceptorship is not:

- the answer to all problems that a newly qualified nurse will face,
- intended to replace mandatory training,
- meant to be a replacement for processes concerning performance management,
- a replacement for processes in place that the NMC uses (or can use) to deal with performance,
- intended to be a further period of training to supplement the undergraduate pre-registration nursing programme,
- formal coaching,
- mentorship,
- statutory or clinical supervision,
- intended to replace induction to employment,
- intended to be done in or completed in isolation.

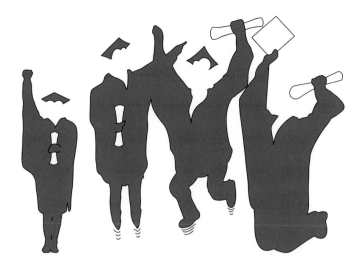

SECTION SUMMARY

Preceptorship guidelines have been produced, but how these are implemented is up to the individual organisations. The NMC has advised that a period of preceptorship should be made available to nurses entering registered practice for the first time. Preceptorship is a period of time that will become the foundation for nurses at the beginning of their nursing career. It does not provide activity that has already been covered as part of the undergraduate nursing programme. Preceptorship is not a tool to manage performance or competence, it is an important activity that you will be engaged with as soon as you qualify as a nurse. In time you will be providing such support to other newly qualified nurses.

As you undertake a programme of preceptorship your confidence will strengthen and you will become an even more autonomous practitioner. You will refine your skills, values and behaviours as you commence your lifelong learning career in the profession of nursing.

Preceptorship framework

The Department of Health (2010) reviewed a number of models and approaches to preceptorship adopted in various other countries and within different professional groups; this included a specific focus on Scotland's multiprofessional preceptorship programme, Flying Start NHS. There is a variety of innovative and creative ways of providing preceptorship programmes (Myrick *et al.*, 2011).

There is a tripartite arrangement associated with preceptorship (see Figure 18.1), and each member of the tripartite partnership has specific responsibilities. Table 18.1 summarises the elements of preceptorship from a variety of perspectives.

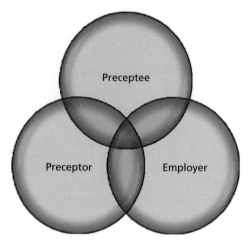

Figure 18.1 The tripartite relationship of preceptorship.

Table 18.1 A summary of the elements of preceptorship

Preceptee	Preceptor	Employer
Chance to apply and develop the knowledge, skills and values previously gained	Duty to develop others professionally to achieve potential	A method of quality assurance
Develop specific competence related to your role	An agent used to formalise and demonstrate continuing professional development	Embeds the Knowledge and Skills Framework at the start of employment (where Knowledge and Skills Frameworks are used)
Access support in implanting the values and expectations of the profession		
Personalised programme of development, including post-registration learning; for example, leadership, management and effectively working within a multidisciplinary team	Responsibility to discuss individual practice and offer feedback	Encourages and fosters an open, honest and transparent culture among staff
	Responsibility to share knowledge and experience	It supports the delivery of high-quality efficient health and social care
Opportunity to reflect on practice and receive feedback		

Preceptee	Preceptor	Employer
Take responsibility for individual learning and development by learning how to 'manage self'	Demonstrate insight and empathy with the newly qualified staff nurse during the transition phase	Articulates the employer's delivery of the NHS Constitution and other key policies
Continuation of lifelong learning	Act as a role model	It indicates the employers commitment to learning
Enables the adoption of the principles of the NHS Constitution	Receive preparation for the role	
	Enables the adoption of the principles of the NHS Constitution	

Source: adapted Department of Health (2010).

 ## Implementing preceptorship

There are a number of learning methods that can be integrated into preceptorship, which enable programmes to be personalised, meeting the needs of each newly registered staff nurse and building their confidence as a practising professional. Effective preceptorship is likely to see the newly registered practitioner engage in a range of activities for varying amounts of time over the first 6–12 months of their first post-registration role. Careful consideration needs to be given to ensuring cost-effective investment of the time and resources devoted to preceptorship to allow a good balance between effective preceptorship and wider provision.

There are no definitive rules or regulations that constitute a best approach. It is important that preceptorship reflects the requirements of the newly qualified staff nurse. The Department of Health (2010) suggests that there are two core components:

- theoretical learning (e.g. classroom-based reading or distance/e-learning),
- supervision/guided reflection on practice (one to one or in a small group, face to face or from a distance).

It is suggested that an optimal mix of these core components should consist of 4–6 days in total for theoretical learning and about 18 hours in total for supervision/guided reflection, but the exact mix will depend on the nurse and the setting in which she/he works. Attention should be paid to the context of the individual's professional responsibilities and the needs of their employer.

Records should be kept for preceptorship; this can be done in line with the requirements of the Knowledge and Skills Framework appraisal process, current continuing professional development requirements and the requirements of the NMC.

Continuing professional development

Continuing professional development (CPD) is the collective name for a range of activities through which you prove your fitness to practise. The Department of Health (2003) suggests that CPD should include a wide range of learning activities through which professionals maintain and develop throughout their career, ensuring that they retain their ability to practise safely, effectively and legally within their evolving scope of practice.

> When I first started my course (in 1997) they said 'this is the first day of the rest of your life. If you think it is all over after 3 years think again; the learning just begins then'. They were spot on. I am now a Matron for acute medicine and I learn something new every single day. *Cecilia, Matron*

Preceptorship, according to the Council of Deans of Health (2009), should be seen as a model of enhancement, acknowledging the new graduate nurse as a safe, competent yet novice practitioner who will continue to develop competence as their career progresses. This is where CPD comes into play.

PEARLS OF WISDOM

C continuing: your learning never ceases regardless of your age or seniority,

P professional: CPD is about professional competence,

D development: it aims to improve your personal performance and enhances career progression.

Clearly there is a close relationship with preceptorship and CPD. You will have already been introduced to the need for lifelong learning and the requirement to ensure that you are professionally developed (Chapter 14 discusses the professional portfolio) as part of your undergraduate nursing programme.

CPD is an NMC requirement, both professionally and legally. Nurses must maintain their registration by meeting the Post Registration Education and Practice (PREP) standards set by the NMC. To stay on the register, nurses must renew their registration every 3 years. This is called periodic renewal. Nurses also pay an annual fee at the end of the first and second year of the registration period. This is called annual retention.

To maintain your registration with the NMC, the PREP standards must be met and you need to declare you have completed:

- 450 hours of registered practice in the previous 3 years, and
- 35 hours of learning activity (CPD) in the previous 3 years.

There are a number of ways that the NMC's practice standards can be met; for example, through administrative, supervisory, teaching, research and managerial roles as well as providing direct patient care (Nursing and Midwifery Council, 2011). If the nurse fails to meet the PREP standards, an approved return-to-practice course must be undertaken before the nurse can renew their registration.

The NMC, like other professional regulators in healthcare (for example, the General Medical Council), periodically reviews and updates its standards for the maintenance and renewal of registration. These reviews form the basis of the NMC's approach to revalidation. It is essential therefore that you keep up to date with any developments in this important area.

How the nurse provides the evidence supporting his or her CPD is a matter of personal choice: there are no hard and fast rules governing this. It must be remembered, however, that as part of its audit requirements the NMC may request and require a nurse to provide evidence of how he or she has maintained their professional development. It is common for a nurse to use a professional portfolio to do this. There are no set conditions as to how it should look; neither is there any prerequisite concerning the content of the portfolio. Professional portfolios are discussed in Chapter 14.

PEARLS OF WISDOM

Remember, it is entirely up to you how you submit evidence to the NMC to show that you are meeting the PREP standards. If you are submitting by portfolio, below is a checklist you may wish to use to ensure that the contents are fit for purpose.

Action	Tick
Is the table of contents clear, with cross-tabulated page numbers?	
Is it well presented and organised?	
Is it user-friendly?	

Action	Tick
Could other people easily navigate their way around it? Do you need to provide more signposts?	
Are you using an assortment of appropriate sources to support your learning?	
Have you used the most suitable media to demonstrate your learning?	
Are you able to give evidence of clear reflective action?	
Is the evidence you are submitting authentic?	
Does the evidence reflect what you claim to have achieved?	
Are the contents true, are they accurate and is this your own work?	
Have you respected confidentiality?	
Is your profile up to date?	

To achieve what is expected of you in terms of CPD you must actively engage in lifelong learning for the rest of your professional life. Lifelong learning is an important feature of maintaining competency in your professional practice.

Post-registration education and practice

Post-registration education and practice (PREP) is a set of standards and guidance produced by the NMC (Nursing and Midwifery Council, 2011) that have been designed to help you provide a high standard of patient care. The PREP standards should always be read in conjunction with the NMC's code of professional conduct (Nursing and Midwifery Council, 2008). There are two elements associated with the standards:

- the PREP (practice) standard,
- the PREP (continuing professional development) standard.

PREP helps nurses demonstrate their ability to be a lifelong learner and to:

- provide a high standard of practice and care,
- keep up to date with new developments in health and social care settings,
- think and reflect for oneself,
- demonstrate keeping up to date and developing their practice,
- demonstrate to the patient and others that they are a knowledgeable, up-to-date practitioner capable of CPD.

PREP cannot guarantee that you are competent, but it is an essential element of clinical governance, affecting all healthcare professionals.

The PREP (practice) standard

To meet the practice standard the nurse must be able to provide evidence that they have undertaken 450 hours in their capacity as a nurse. You will only be deemed to have met the practice standard for nursing by practising nursing. Table 18.2 outlines ways in which you can meet the practice element of the PREP standard.

Table 18.2 Ways which the practice element of the PREP (practice) standard can be met

In paid work	When employed by an organisation such as an NHS Trust, a care home, an independent healthcare provider, a nursing agency, a health authority or health board, an educational institution or another type of company or organisation, or if working in independent practice
In unpaid work	When working on a voluntary basis in a role that requires registration; for example, an established healthcare charity
When not working	When taking a career break within the 3 year re-registration period, the nurse may still be able to meet the practice standard if he or she has completed the required hours in practice as a registered nurse at some stage during those 3 years. If the nurse does not meet the PREP (practice) standard, an approved return-to-practice course will need to be undertaken and successfully completed prior to the nurse being able to renew their registration.

Source: adapted Nursing and Midwifery Council (2011).

 The PREP (continuing professional development) standard

The PREP (continuing professional development) standard demands you undertake some form of CPD. See Box 18.1 that outlines the elements of this standard.

Box 18.1 The PREP (continuing professional development) standard

- Undertake at least 35 hours of learning activity applicable to your practice during the 3 years before renewal of your registration
- Compile a personal professional profile of your learning activity
- Act in accordance with any request from the NMC to audit how these requirements have been met

Source: adapted Nursing and Midwifery Council (2011).

The learning activity that you undertake to meet this standard has to be relevant to your practice. There is, however, no such thing as an approved PREP (continuing professional development) learning activity. In your professional profile you must document (by whichever method you choose) your relevant learning activity and the ways in which this has informed and influenced your nursing practice.

ACTIVITY 18.4

Consider your future CPD needs: what do you think they may be? How will you achieve them? Are there any potential barriers to achieving them and, if so, how will you overcome them? If a fee is required to meet those needs, who will pay it?

The NMC has provided guidance for recording your PREP (continuing professional development) learning. You should document each learning activity that you have undertaken in the 3 years prior to renewing your registration. You need to think about how you might record what you do, what you learn and how you apply it to your professional practice.

The record should provide a list as well as a description of your workplace or organisation and role for the last 3 years. Record your workplace(s) and your work or role(s) that relate to the learning activity that you are describing. If you have worked in various places, but in essentially the same role (for example, if you are a bank nurse or an agency nurse), you can group this type of work together, summarising it in this section.

Identify the nature of the learning activity, and what it was that you did. You should record the learning activity related to the work you have identified for the last 3 years, stating the date or period when this activity took place and how many hours the learning activity took you to complete.

Describe the learning activity: what did it consist of? Provide a detailed description of the activity, what it was that made you decide to undertake that specific learning or how the opportunity arose, where, when and how you did the learning, and what it was that you expected to gain from doing it. How did the learning relate to your work, and what was the outcome? You are advised to record the effect it has had on the way in which you work or how you intend to work in the future, and any follow-up learning that you may be thinking about in the future.

PEARLS OF WISDOM

You might want to think about concluding the description with 'The ways in which this learning has influenced my work are ...'.

SECTION SUMMARY

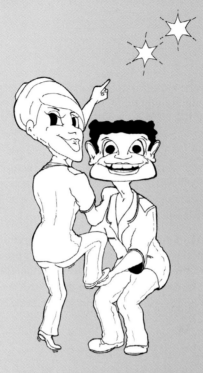

CPD for nurses is a legal requirement. The NMC requires that you meet two standards before you are able to register or renew your licence to practice: a CPD standard and a practice standard. You may be required to provide evidence that reflects your ability to meet the standards. The way you provide your evidence is up to you. The most common method of doing this is with a professional portfolio. Failure to meet the standards may necessitate a return-to-practice programme of study. Fabrication of facts (fraud) can lead to allegations of professional misconduct.

CPD provides a means by which nurses are able to maintain their knowledge and skills and develop clinical and academic qualities in their professional lives. It is the explicit updating of professional knowledge and the improvement of professional competence throughout the nurse's working life. CPD is a commitment to being professional, keeping up to date and continuously seeking to improve.

The NMC reviews its approach to CPD and the PREP standards in a periodic fashion, as do other health and social care professions. This makes it important that you keep up to date on current requirements.

I just can't wait to get out and put into practice all that I have learned over the these last 3 years. I will have my feet firmly on the ground but my head will be way up in the clouds.
Bina, third year student

 ## Summary

The public have a right to expect that the nurse caring for them is competent and up to date with contemporary practice. Preceptorship and the need to undertake CPD are ways in which the NMC can reassure the public of this. Although preceptorship and the need to provide evidence of CPD may seem to be some years away in the eyes of a student, for new graduates it is an imminent reality as their name is entered on the professional register. Professional registration is just one step, and you must be deemed competent at the point of entry and as you notify the NMC of your intention to practice. This means that you have to be a lifelong learner, developing skills, knowledge and attitudes.

CPD provides a means by which nurses are able to maintain their knowledge and skills and develop clinical and academic qualities in their professional lives. It is the explicit updating of professional knowledge and the improvement of professional competence throughout the nurse's working life. CPD is a commitment to being professional, keeping up to date and seeking continuously to improve.

 ## References

Broad, P., Walker, J., Boden, R. and Barnes, A. (2011) Developing a 'model of transition' prior to preceptorship. *British Journal of Nursing* 20(20), 1298–1301

Council of Deans of Health (2009) *Report From the Preceptorship Workshops Retreat.* Unpublished report, 27 May 2009. Council of Deans of Health, Bristol

Department of Health (2003) *Allied Health Professions Project: Demonstrating Competence Through Continuing Professional Development (CPD) – Final Report.* www.dh.gov.uk/prod_consum_dh/groups/dh_digitalassets/@dh/@en/documents/digitalasset/dh_4071462.pdf

Department of Health (2008) *A High Quality Workforce: NHS Next Stage Review.* Department of Health, London.

Department of Health (2010) *Preceptorship Framework for Newly Registered Nurses, Midwives and Allied Health Professionals.* Department of Health, London

Kramer, M. (1974) *Reality Shock: Why Nurses Leave Nursing.* Mosby, St Louis, MO

Myrick, F., Caplan, W., Smitten, J. and Rusk, K. (2011) Preceptorship/mentor education: a world of possibilities through e – learning technology. *Nurse Education Today* 31(310), 263–7

National Nursing Research Unit (2009) *Providing Preceptorship for Newly Qualified Nurses: What are the Components of Success?* www.kcl.ac.uk/content/1/c6/04/96/09/PolicyIssue16.pdf

Nursing and Midwifery Council (2006) *Preceptorship Guidelines.* NMC Circular 21/2006. Nursing and Midwifery Council, London

Nursing and Midwifery Council (2008) *The Code: Standards of Conduct, Performance and Ethics for Nurses and Midwives.* Nursing and Midwifery Council, London

Nursing and Midwifery Council (2010) *Standards for Pre registration Nursing Education*. http://standards.nmc-uk.org/PublishedDocuments/Standards%20for%20pre-registration%20nursing%20education%2016082010.pdf

Nursing and Midwifery Council (2011) *The Prep Handbook*. www.nmc-uk.org/Documents/Standards/NMC_Prep-handbook_2011.pdf

 # Resources

Flying Start England

www.flyingstartengland.nhs.uk/

Flying Start England is the national development programme for all newly qualified nurses, midwives and allied health professionals in NHS England. It is designed to support the transition from student to newly qualified health professional by supporting learning in everyday practice through a range of learning activities.

Flying Start Scotland

www.flyingstart.scot.nhs.uk/

Flying Start is the core programme for all staff to support induction, transition and the NHS Knowledge and Skills Framework development review cycle in Scotland. This resource is excellent and provides much information and help when you become a newly qualified staff nurse.

Positive Thinking Principles

www.positive-thinking-principles.com/action-plan-template.html

This site provides an action plan template that you can use to set your own personal goals using a SMART approach (the website explains what this acronym means).

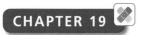

CHAPTER 19

What Do I Do If . . .? Questions You Did Not Want To Ask Out Loud

- Questions, queries and concerns that students have had
- Where possible, answers are provided

Nurses make up the largest talent pool in health and social care. They provide 24-hour care 365 days a year and make vital contributions to individuals, families and communities. Nurses touch those they care for and they are touched by the people to whom they offer care. Usually this in a positive manner but there are times when things go wrong and the relationship can cause harm. Thankfully, these incidents are few and far between.

As a nurse you will meet a lot of very different people, and there will be some whose values and beliefs will clash with your own, some who will like you and some who will take a dislike to you (do remember this is not about you, it is about the patient, first and foremost). You are going to meet people who are rich and some who are poor, those who are clean and others who are dirty, some people will be intelligent and there will be some not so intelligent, some will be sophisticated, elegant and articulate and others will not. The one thing that they all have in common is they are people, all of whom should be afforded the same respect, attention, compassion and care.

As you move closer to putting the initials RN after your name you may have many questions on your mind, but which you not yet wanted to speak out loud. This final chapter looks at some of these questions and aims to provide answers where possible. The format of this chapter is different to that of the others: it uses some of the chapter headings from the book as a structure. The questions are real-life ones that students have raised with me in the past.

The Student Nurse Toolkit: An Essential Guide for Surviving Your Course, First Edition. Ian Peate.
© 2013 John Wiley & Sons, Ltd. Published 2013 by John Wiley & Sons, Ltd.

Entry to nursing

I have a criminal conviction and I am not sure if they will even invite me to interview: should I declare it?

You should declare your criminal conviction.

Declaration of criminal convictions, including spent convictions, verbal cautions and bind-over orders demonstrates the university's intention to reduce the risk of harm or injury to patients, families, students and staff caused by any criminal behaviour of students. The university must know about any convictions that you have. If you declare a criminal conviction your application will be assessed according to the published selection criteria for the programme you have selected. The NMC require the university to have processes and procedures in place to manage students who have a criminal conviction (Nursing and Midwifery Council, 2010a).

Information relating to your conviction will be considered separately from your academic achievements by appointed university staff. Information disclosed by you about a criminal conviction will only be passed to the university's Criminal Convictions Group (or equivalent); this is a specified group of appointed staff and usually includes clinicians.

The university may want to ask you for more information prior to a decision being made. Third parties may also be approached for information, but this will not be done unless you give your permission. If you are charged with a relevant criminal offence after you have submitted your application, or after you have been made an offer, you must inform the university as soon as possible. When you do this, the same process as for convictions declared at the time of applying will be carried out as described.

If you fail to declare a relevant criminal conviction at any point in the admission process your application will be considered to be fraudulent and the university will retain the right to withdraw your application. If you have been made an offer by the university then the university may in these circumstances withdraw or amend the offer made. If you have been admitted as a student you may be subject to disciplinary action and this could result in your expulsion from the university.

Criminal Records Bureau check

Those applying to study nursing are exempt under the Rehabilitation of Offenders Act 1974 and as such the university and prospective employers are entitled to ask exempted questions. All applicants to nursing and health-related programmes are required to undergo a formal Criminal Records Bureau (CRB) check. The CRB check may be carried out on an annual basis; each university has its own procedures in place for this.

In Scotland a similar system is in place. Disclosure Scotland provides organisations with criminal history information.

Data protection

All records and correspondence relating to your declaration of a relevant criminal conviction will be securely stored in accordance with the university's data protection policy. If you have declared a criminal conviction and your application is successful, all records and correspondence relating to your application and supporting materials will form part of your personal record and will be kept in the same way as all other student records. However, any information relating to your conviction will be stored separately and securely. A decision will be made, based upon your particular circumstances and informed by the recommendation of the university, on who, if anyone, in the university (and clinical practice) should be provided with further details of your conviction. If your application is successful you will be provided with further information on data retention.

If you have declared a criminal conviction and your application is unsuccessful, any paper copies of information relating to your conviction will be shredded immediately. Your consent should always be obtained before seeking further information about any declared convictions from third parties.

While on your programme of study the NMC (Nursing and Midwifery Council, 2010b) notes that the behaviour and conduct of students in their personal life may also have an impact on their fitness to practise, their ability to complete their programme of study and the willingness of the university to sign the declaration of good health and good character. Inappropriate behaviour may include:

- aggressive, violent or threatening behaviour,
- cheating,
- plagiarism,
- misuse of the Internet and social networking sites.

Nurse education: the standards for pre-registration nurse education

I have dyslexia

The Scottish Government, Dyslexia Scotland and the Cross Party Group on Dyslexia in the Scottish Parliament have provided the following definition of dyslexia; this is only one of many definitions available.

> Dyslexia can be described as a continuum of difficulties in learning to read, write and/or spell, which persist despite the provision of appropriate learning opportunities. These difficulties often do not reflect a person's cognitive abilities and may not be typical of performance in other areas. The impact of dyslexia as a barrier to learning varies in degree (Scottish Government, 2012).

Under the terms of the Disability Discrimination Act 1995 dyslexia is considered to be a disability and dyslexic health professionals are therefore entitled to receive 'reasonable adjustments' in both the educational institution and the workplace. Reasonable adjustments enable disabled students to participate on an equal basis with other students. A full understanding of the individual's profile is necessary to offer the most effective support, and when this has been carried out reasonable adjustments will be put in place. However, the student must demonstrate that they are fit to practice and meet all the learning competencies and skills in the same way as others.

If you have been diagnosed with dyslexia you will be invited to make that known prior to commencing your programme of study. It is essential to remember that an individual with dyslexia is likely to need ongoing and possibly increasing support as their programme of study progresses. The university has a duty to make reasonable adjustments to help you with your studies. If you think you may have dyslexia then this should be discussed with your personal tutor in the first instance.

Dyslexia affects people in different ways and symptoms range from mild to severe. Strategies that might work for one student in a placement setting may not be helpful for another and because of this an individual assessment of your needs will be made usually by a nominated, experienced member of staff, called a disability adviser. Support is available but you need to make known your needs and as you access that support you may feel more confident about disclosing your disability. You have a right to confidentiality about your disability, and you must be aware that if you limit your disclosure you restrict the reasonable adjustments that can be implemented.

 ## The NMC and other regulatory bodies

 ### When I qualify what do I have to do to register with the NMC?

The university will notify the NMC of your success. You will be sent an application pack once the NMC have received your course completion details from the university. It usually takes 7–10 working days for the pack to reach you by post. The university is also required to send the NMC a declaration of good health and good character form, so be sure that the university has up-to-date records of your personal details. When you return your application form to the NMC you will also be required to pay a fee.

You have to ensure that your application form is completed correctly. Before sending it check that:

- your student PIN is entered correctly,
- your course details are entered correctly,
- your clearly state which part of the register you are applying for,
- your personal details are correct (for example, name, address, date of birth),

- ☙ your university has the same details for you as does the NMC: it can delay your registration if the NMC has to check this,
- ☙ you pay the correct amount, and remember to sign the cheque,
- ☙ you send your cheque and forms together,
- ☙ you complete and send the declaration of good health and good character with everything else.

You have to apply to register within 5 years of your course completion date. When the NMC has received all of your details your registration will be completed in 2–10 working days. You will receive a statement of entry 7–10 days after you are registered. There are times when it can take the NMC a little longer: if you have not heard anything from them within 3 weeks then call them.

The university

What if I fail an assignment?

Failing a module can come as quite a shock for some people. Students do fail assignments and should this happen to you there are a number of people who can help and support you. Your peers will be there for you along with the teaching staff, helping you through it and providing encouragement. You may feel like the world had ended, but seek support, resubmit and try to pass at the next attempt.

You need to be aware that you are individually responsible for managing your own study and undertaking all assessments in the format required and at the time specified. It is therefore important that you make every effort to become familiar with the university's policies and regulations concerning assessments. They can be really complex but understanding them will give you a head start.

If you have received your results and you have not passed all of your work then you need to adhere to university regulations with regards to process; you may need to attend an advice and guidance session (it is usual at these sessions that you agree your programme and modules for next year to ensure a smooth return to your studies). Be sure you understand what the key dates are in respect to referral; for example, the dates of the resit examination period. Make sure you understand the deadlines and whether the work is to be submitted manually or online. This is important, so check it with your module tutor (or the equivalent).

If you are sending referred coursework by mail then it is strongly recommended that you post it using some form of recorded delivery. All work must be posted in advance of the deadline to allow time for delivery; it is very important that you keep your receipt and obtain proof of the date and time of posting. Your work must arrive by the deadline.

If you have failed the first 'sit' for any of your modules you may be permitted to resit, but remember that it is not an automatic right. When you receive your results list this will tell you which modules you are required to resit, if any, and whether you have to resit coursework or assessment under controlled conditions, or both. Reassessment details together with the dates for resits and resubmissions are usually contained in your module handbook.

You are strongly advised to speak to the members of staff for the modules you have to resit to find out what has gone wrong and what remedial work you will be required to do.

Retakes (reassessment)

Every 'attempt' at a module includes a 'sit' and a 'resit'. On occasion you may be given an exceptional retake of a module following a sit and resit if you have had extenuating circumstances accepted or at the discretion of the Award Board, which will take into account your modular profile (your academic history). You will be required to re-enrol before you can undertake any further assessment and this means you will have to complete paperwork. The student centre (or equivalent) can help you with this.

You may have to pay a resit charge. You are strongly advised to consult your personal tutor and/or programme leader about arrangements for re-enrolling for a second or subsequent attempt at a module.

Practice learning opportunities

I have never seen a dead body and I am anxious about it

Your anxiety is understandable. Death is an emotive subject. Most people have little direct or personal experience of it and because of this we can often be ignorant or afraid of death and dying. You are not alone if this is how you feel.

There are many ways in which we can respond to death and often it depends on our relationship to the dying person. We might react quite differently to the death of a child as opposed to the death of an older person. We may be affected by the sudden death of a person more than an expected death.

Knowing or being made aware of what to expect may ease any fear of what you might see and experience. Speaking with staff on your clinical placement about your anxiety and discussing it with your personal tutor may help you. Some people find it easier to speak to a minister of faith, for example a rabbi, imam or priest. There are no hard-and-fast rules as to who you can talk to, just as there are no easy answers to help with the fears or anxieties you have. Acknowledging that you have these anxieties is a step in the right direction.

You might want to consider this issue as a topic for reflection. Reflecting on your feelings may help you. The first death you experience will be something that stays with you throughout your life, so it is a significant experience and not one to be shooed away.

I am being bullied at university

Just because bullying in universities is not spoken about does not mean that it is not happening. Bullying does occur in universities. There are many reasons why students do not report bullying. Sometimes they do not trust the university services that are there to help them deal with bullying, and feel that nothing will be done about it. Students may find it difficult to speak of their ordeal; this might be due to embarrassment or the inability to self-admit. Being bullied has the potential to ruin your university course and your nursing career. Confiding in somebody – your personal tutor, the student union, university counselling services or occupational health – can help you, and there are processes in place that can help you deal with such circumstances.

Do not keep it to yourself. Keep a diary of the events that have caused upset (when, where, any witnesses, what time it happened and the impact it had on you) and then take it to members of staff. If you feel they are not prepared to do anything about it, take it to the Dean of Faculty.

Common myths and misconceptions about bullying include:

- there is no bullying here,
- bullying toughens you up,
- you have to stand up for yourself,
- just ignore it and it will go away,
- it is part of life and you just have to accept it.

Bullying is about impact, not about intent; if you are upset by it then it is not funny, it is no joke.

I have never seen a cardiac arrest and I am just finishing my third year

Some people can go through their whole nursing careers and never see a cardiac arrest. The main thing is to ensure that you are as up to date as you possibly can be. Attend all updates and keep practising the drill. Cardiac arrest is sudden and can occur anywhere at any time, so it may just be a question of time. Hopefully you will never see one.

Managing self

I think I am stressed

Some stress or pressure can be valuable, as it can be what keeps us interested and can permit us to keep up the momentum. Yet, excessive pressure or stress has the potential to lead to stress that damage your health and well-being. Stress can affect anyone at any time. Nurses often find it difficult to recognise and identify that they are suffering from stress as they are too busy caring for others.

Stress appears in many different ways. It is the body's way of alerting you to a threat or a problem. Table 19.1 provides some examples of the symptoms of stress.

Table 19.1 Some symptoms of stress

Physical	Tight chest, racing heart, high blood pressure, headaches, chest pains, nausea, insomnia, sweaty palms, itching, abdominal cramps, drop in immune system, indigestion, ulcers, faster breathing, 'butterflies' in your stomach, dry mouth
Thoughts	Not being able to switch off, lack of attention, feeling disorganised, losing self-esteem, lack of control, poor memory, lack of motivation, lack of sense of humour
Feelings	Loss of confidence, irritability, feeling more emotional, moody, anxious, depressed, panic, restlessness
Behaviour	Increased illness, sickness absence from work, poor relationships, withdrawing, increased consumption of alcohol/nicotine/drugs/food, loss of appetite, carelessness, violence, aggressive behaviour, blaming others, swearing

You must remember that we all experience the symptoms of stress in different ways. The list of symptoms outlined in Table 19.1 is not exhaustive and your experience may be different from those that are listed in the table. One person may find some things easy to cope with but another person may find the same things stressful. The important thing to note is that your experience is no less valid: all it indicates is that we all experience things differently.

 Coping with stress

Here are some simple steps that you might want to take to help you manage the stress you are experiencing. These measures can help you enhance your ability to cope with a stressful situation and enable you to evaluate matters differently, helping you to put things into a different perspective. Some examples might include the following.

- Take enjoyable exercise: exercise can burn up excess adrenaline and release endorphins (these are the feel-good hormones). You do not necessarily have to be at the gym for hours if this is not what you enjoy. You might want to take up gardening, or take regular walks, go for a gentle swim, take an exercise class, or engage in more competitive sports such as netball, football or tennis.
- Avoid harmful substances, for example, tobacco, alcohol or drugs: these have the ability to lead you to feel more stressed and unable to cope. They can bring an immediate sense of relief, but this is short term and will not allow you to learn to cope with the stresses experienced. They can make the

situation worse, preventing you from putting things into perspective and remaining rational.

 Learn to relax: when you engage in relaxation this communicates to your brain that the threat has gone, allowing you to recharge your batteries. If you do not already have a hobby think about taking up something that has previously interested you. Relaxation can also come about by listening to music or by having a long soak in the bath. There are many relaxation CDs available that could help you learn relaxation skills if you are finding it difficult to relax.

 Don't bottle it up: it really is good to talk. Talk to someone close to you. It can be helpful to speak to someone about how you are feeling; it can give you a different perspective on things. If you find it difficult to talk about your emotions to those who are close to you then try writing about them instead.

The portfolio

I am applying for my first staff nurse post

This is where the professional portfolio comes to the fore. Make sure it is up to date and that the content makes you stand out from the crowd. When you have seen a job you are keen on make sure that you have the skills to match the requirements. When undergraduate programmes of study end (sometimes this occurs twice a year, usually in September or February) there are usually a great number of students applying for jobs, so do not be too disappointed if you do not get the job you have applied for. Take each opportunity to learn from the whole experience: seeking the job out, submission of the application and, if you are invited for interview, the interview itself. You can also learn from any feedback the interviewers provide you with.

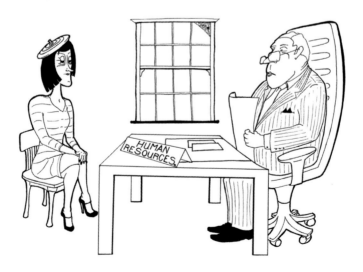

It is always advisable that you start looking for a job 2–3 months before your programme is due to finish, although there is no consensus on when it is best to apply. Preparation is the best way to get the job you want. Preparation really does show through, both when your application is being considered for the shortlist and at interview, when you are in front of a panel. As part of that preparation you should always request an informal visit, regardless of whether you have been working or are working in the care area you are applying for. The informal visit provides you with an opportunity to view the job from the perspective of a staff nurse rather than a student nurse.

You should be up to date with contemporary issues in the areas of heath and social care. Make yourself aware of local and national politics demonstrates insight as well as enthusiasm.

Your CV and the application form are the first things the panel will see of you. They may not want to invite you to interview if these essential documents are poorly presented, so you must make every effort to ensure the information and the presentation are complete, with no gaps. Presentation and content are really important here.

You may be required to complete the application form online. Beware that there may not be an option for a spellcheck so take care and ensure that your spelling, grammar and syntax are correct. It is a good idea to include a covering letter, which provides an introduction and makes a good first impression. The covering letter is your chance to tell the panel why you are a great fit for the job and passionate about being given an opportunity to prove yourself. If you do not include a covering letter the panel (or the person shortlisting) has to scan read your CV, which takes time, to try to determine whether you have the right skills and experience for the position.

Be sure that you pay attention to your referees, and that they match the requirements (sometimes the employer insists on the inclusion of a lecturer). It is a common courtesy to ask your prospective referees in advance whether they are willing to provide a reference.

Be on time, all the time. It may seem like a no-brainer, but how can you expect to be considered seriously for a job if you arrive late to the interview? Even being a couple of minutes late sends out the wrong message: it signals to the panel that work is where you would rather not be. Show that you are keen by showing up at least 10–15 minutes early, with time to spare to get settled before the interview.

Dress for success: image really is everything. If you want to be considered as a professional, then you have to dress like one. This might appear shallow but your appearance is a visual cue to the employer as to what type of employee you will be. Dress like you already are a professional.

Go the extra mile by learning as much as possible about the job and also about the organisation. Find out as much as you can about the position you are applying for (the informal visit is an ideal opportunity to delve deeper) and where the organisation is going in terms of its business.

Policies, procedures and legal matters

I have been asked to write a statement on the ward where I work

It is inevitable that during the course of your career as a nurse you will be asked to produce a statement. There are number of different types of statements and you should always seek advice from your personal tutor, link lecturer or trade union prior to writing a statement. Here are some key recommendations and suggestions for preparing a statement.

The statement can be a written report about a patient or it might be requested from a witness or someone involved in an incident that is under investigation. The various types of statement have specific purposes and effects. A police statement, for example, could result in you giving evidence in criminal proceedings or to a coroner. A statement that is made under caution may later be used as evidence in criminal proceedings. You cannot be forced to make a statement if it criminally implicates you.

Nurses have a duty to assist in investigations (Nursing and Midwifery Council, 2008) and all employees have an implied duty to conform to any reasonable request by their employer. If you are asked to comment on a particular patient or their care, remember that confidentiality rules mean you cannot generally disclose the identity of the patient or relatives.

You could also be asked to make a statement as a witness to an incident that you were not directly involved in. This may include, for example, witnessing a patient assaulting a colleague. This could lead to formal proceedings against another person, and you may be required to attend a disciplinary or grievance hearing.

Preparing to write a statement

Preparing and writing a statement requires a lot of thought, time and consideration. You must take time in preparation to ensure that the final version is accurate, clear, concise and relevant. Prior to writing your statement be sure what is required of you and ensure that you have all the necessary information and resources to hand. Consider the following.

- Requests for a statement should be in writing so that you understand exactly what you are being asked to write. If the request is made verbally then you should ask for the request to be confirmed in writing.
- Agree a time frame to complete the statement: good statements can often take longer to write than you might think.

- If you are required to write a statement in connection with a potential legal action you are strongly advised to seek advice: again, speak to your personal tutor, link lecturer or trade union.
- Never reveal patients' and relatives' identities; for example, use 'patient X' throughout the statement.
- State your position (i.e. second year, mental health student nurse) and the basis for the statement. State what is your personal recollection and what can be corroborated as fact, with reference to healthcare records, reports, clinical guidelines or standards.
- Relate the facts from the beginning and maintain strict chronological order, giving precise dates and times. Be clear about the times you were on and off duty on the days in question and about what you saw and heard.
- Do not make the assumption that the reader knows anything about the case. The statement will therefore be a factual 'story' which tells the reader the circumstances of an incident as you remember them.
- Avoid general statements such as 'routine observations were made'.
- Do not speculate, elaborate or exaggerate.
- Remember that you could be challenged on the content and details of your account.
- Hearsay is second-hand, rather than first-hand, evidence (for example: 'I heard Sean say that he had seen Marie give the injection'). Only relate what you were told.
- Write your statement in simple terms, avoiding jargon or official language, and be as brief as possible, covering all the essential points.
- Avoid emotional language.
- Include references to documents, papers, books or notes if relevant.
- Always sign your statement, giving your full name and job title below your signature, together with the date on which it was signed. Remember to keep a copy.

Statement format

Table 19.2 provides an overview of how a statement may be structured.

Table 19.2 Suggested structure of a statement

General format	All pages must be numbered
	There should be clear, wide margins at each side.
	Number all paragraphs; they should be short, precise and no more than six lines long. Paragraphs should have subject headings, where appropriate.
	Use double spacing
	Write in the first person (i.e. I, me)
	Have your statement typed or use plain white A4 paper, writing neatly in black ink or ballpoint pen

Front page	Your name
	Your occupation or job title
	Your professional address (i.e. the university)
	Subject of statement (e.g. patient/client X at what incident/ location)
Introduction	'I am a student nurse at [insert your university]. I am in [cite your year of study and your field]. My previous experience includes....'
	'This statement is based on [personal recollection/review of records or combination].'
	'I have been involved in the care of patient X since [date].'
	'I am responding to a request for a written statement.'
The body (narrative)	Explain the event, incident or accident in chronological order. Use subheadings and new paragraphs to structure your statement, for example:
	☒ response to allegations (1, 2, 3, etc.),
	☒ informal meetings,
	☒ telephone calls.
Summary or closing statement	Recap the main points, and avoid adding new information or comments.
Statement of truth	'This statement is true to the best of my knowledge and belief.'
	Your signature and title
	Date
	If you have had any help writing the statement state 'I have prepared this statement with the assistance of [name of person, job title, contact details]'.

Source: adapted Royal College of Nursing (2011).

Always keep a copy of your statement for future reference. You should have any statement you prepare checked by your personal tutor, link lecturer or trade union before you submit it.

 ## Preceptorship and continuing professional development

 ### I am due to start my new job in a few weeks time and I am really nervous about the first day

You are a registered nurse, you have undergone a 3-year educational programme of study to prepare you for this job and you have been deemed competent to practise nursing. There would be something wrong if you did not have some anxiety about your first day at work as a staff nurse. Starting any job is a time that can be filled with opportunity, hope and anticipation; it can also be tainted with insecurity and doubt. There are many people around who want you to suceed, helping you keep clear of potential slip-ups and offering you tried-and-tested strategies that can help with a smooth transition to your new and exciting environment. Here are some tips that you may find useful when starting your new job.

- Take every opportunity to learn.
- Speak up if you do not know or you are unsure.
- Do not ever be afraid to ask questions or to question.
- Work closely with your preceptor to share in her or his wisdom. If you are not getting on with him or her, speak to them about it and if things do not improve then speak with your manager. When the formal period of preceptorship ends, seek out informal mentors.
- Try to steer clear of unhealthy dynamics when you are new to the job and trying to fit in. Avoid politics, gossip and back biting: it will sap your energy levels.
- Apply all of the knowledge gained in nursing school to being a productive team member, a team player; offer to help others during difficult situations. Get to know the people you work with (this is not just the nurses but the other people without whom the service would not function). Acknowledge them and their expertise.
- Be alert, watch how others you work with manage situations, people and care needs: watch the experts at work. Ask more senior people how they do things and how they would manage certain situations.
- Take time out to care for yourself and make your own needs known.
- Acknowledge that change can be scary, but do not be so hard on yourself when you get frustrated or discouraged. It takes time to feel a part of the team, to feel confident and to adapt to the transition from student to staff nurse.

 ## Summary

This final chapter has provided you with some answers to some of the questions you may have had. It may not have answered them as fully as you might have wanted, but it is a start. There are many resources, human and material, that are available to help you, but you have to ask the questions in order to get the answers. Remember that very soon you will be the person people come to with their own questions.

 ## References

Nursing and Midwifery Council (2008) *The Code: Standards of Conduct, Performance and Ethics for Nurses and Midwives.* Nursing and Midwifery Council, London

Nursing and Midwifery Council (2010a) *Standards for Pre registration Nursing Education.* http://standards.nmc-uk.org/PublishedDocuments/Standards%20for%20pre-registration%20nursing%20education%2016082010.pdf

Nursing and Midwifery Council (2010b) *Guidance on Professional Conduct for Nursing and Midwifery Students*, 2nd edn. Nursing and Midwifery Council, London

Royal College of Nursing (2011) *Statement Writing*. www.rcn.org.uk/__data/assets/pdf_file/0012/489495/Statement_writing_-_Advice_guide_Final_V3_2.pdf

Scottish Government (2012) "Definition of Dyslexia" www.scotland.gov.uk/Topics/Education/Schools/welfare/ASL/dyslexia

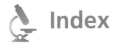

Index

Note: page numbers in *italics* refer to figures, those in **bold** refer to tables, summaries and boxes

abbreviations use 168–9, **170**
  documentation 241, 242–3
  multiple meaning 168–9, **169**
  protocols 251
  records 241, 242–3
abdomen
  anatomical landmarks 171, **172**
  quadrants *171*
  regions 172
abuse *54*, 55
  concerns 55, 57
Access to Medical Reports Act (1988) 244
acronym use 169, 242
action plans 224–5
adult nursing **33**
  practice learning opportunities **120**
  professional values **40**
Adults with Incapacity (Scotland) Act
  (2000) 265
advanced directives 264
advocacy 56
Age of Legal Capacity (Scotland) Act
  (1991) 264
alcohol use 305–6
anatomical landmarks
  abdomen 171, **172**
  terminology 170–2
anatomical planes 170–1
anecdotal evidence **186**
anisocoria **76**
anxieties
  practice learning opportunities 303
  starting new job 310–11
application forms for jobs 307
approved education institution (AEI) 100

assertiveness skills **159**
assessment, practice learning
    opportunities 123–4, **125**
assessment tools 65–77
  Glasgow Coma Scale 73–6
  Malnutrition Universal Screening
    Tool 66–9
  Modified Early Warning Score 69–73
  track-and-trigger scoring system 69,
    70, 71, 72
  Waterlow pressure ulcer assessment
    tool 65–6
assumptions 145
attitudes 145
AVPU scale **72**, 75

battery allegations 262
behaviour
  inappropriate 300
  see also professional conduct
beliefs
  patients 298
  personal of nurses 144–5, **146–7**
best interests
  consent in emergency situations 261
  people without capacity 266
Beveridge Report (1942) 47, **48**
blended learning 111
body mass index (BMI) 67, *68*
Bolam test 257
Bolitho v City and Hackney Health
    Authority [1997] 257
boundaries 147
breach of duty 256, 257–8
Briggs Committee (1970) 29

The Student Nurse Toolkit: An Essential Guide for Surviving Your Course, First Edition. Ian Peate.
© 2013 John Wiley & Sons, Ltd. Published 2013 by John Wiley & Sons, Ltd.

British Association for Parenteral and
        Enteral Nutrition (BAPEN)
        66, **69**
bullying 304
burden of proof, negligence 258

calculations 94–5
capacity 260
    consent **260**, 264–5
    decision making 266
    exceptions to 260–1
    mental health acts 265–6
    minors 264
    presumption of 266
cardiac arrest 304
care 82–3
    documentation in good nursing care
        promotion 235
    environment 116–17
    essential skills clusters **81**, 82–3
        organisational aspects 89, **90**
    integrated care pathway 32
    organisational aspects 89, **90**
    reasonable care standard 254
    refusal by patient 257
    see also quality of care
Care and Compassion (Parliamentary
        and Health Service Ombudsman,
        2011) 83
care providers 52
Care Quality Commission (CQC) 15
careers 1–2
    clinical academic careers 268,
        276–9
    education 274
    entrepreneurship 275
    flexible pathways 275
    housing 274
    independent sector 274
    key elements 271
    leadership 274–5
    modern nursing 271–5, **276**
    modernising 276
    schools 274
    senior clinical roles 272
    social services 274
    structure 273, **273–4**, 274–5
    transferrable skills 269–70
    voluntary sector 274

carers 47
    involvement 270
    unsupported 55
case report **186**
case-controlled study **186**
cataract surgery **76**
charge nurses 272
children, legal capacity 264
children's nursing **33**
    handover of patients 164
    practice learning opportunities
        119, 120
    professional values **40**
chronic illness *see* long-term conditions
CINAHL (Cumulative Index to Nursing and
        Allied Health Literature)
        183, 187
citizenship 49
clinical academic careers 268, 276–9
    benefits of academic roles 277–8
    Department of Health outline of
        aspirations 276, **277**
    knowledge advancement 278
    model framework 278
    resources 278
    role descriptors 278
    skills development 278
    sustainable 275
Clinical Academic Research Career (CARC)
        Framework 276
clinical competence *see* competence
clinical decisions, evidence base
        185, **187**
clinical guidelines *see* guidelines
clinical nurse specialists 272
clinical pathways 250
clinical placement 116
Cochrane Database of Systematic Reviews
        (CDSR) 190
Cochrane Library **183**, 187
*The Code: Standards of Conduct,
        Performance and Ethics for Nurses
        and Midwives see* Nursing and
        Midwifery Council (NMC), code of
        professional conduct
cohort study **186**
Commission for the Future of Nursing
        (2010) 275
commissioning 52

communication 82–6, **88**
  body movements *86*
  channels **156**
  consent 263
  context **156**
  effective 83
  feedback **156**
  handover of patients 164
  haptic 85–6
  learned cultural standards 85
  message **155**
  modifiers 85
  noise **155**
  nonverbal 84–6, 155, **155–6**
  personal space 85, 86
  process 83
  records for facilitation 235
  setting 85
  skills 155, **155–6**
  terminology **170**
  types 84–6
  verbal 84, *86*, 155, **155–6**
community matrons 272
community nurse, handover of
      patients 164
community-based care 117, 269
compassion 80, 82–3
competence
  assessment 124
  definition 38
  development 290
  duty of care 254
  professional portfolio for
      documentation 212, 215
  registered nurses 256, 283
  student nurses 283
competency framework 37–9, **40**
  domains 39, **40**
complaints
  consent 262
  investigation 231
conduct standards 21–2
confidentiality 88, **89**
  disability 301
  duty of care 254
  handover of patients 165
  maintaining 86–7
  professional portfolio 212–13, 223
  records/record keeping 244

reflective writing 209
  statement writing 309
consciousness
  altered 74
  level 74, 75
consent 260–6
  battery allegations 262
  capacity **260**, 260–1, 264–5
  communication 263
  complaints 262
  emergency situations 261
  by implication 263
  informed **260**
  interpreters 263
  language issues 263
  legal proceedings 262
  mental health acts 265–6
  minors (under 16 years) 264
  obtaining 261–2
  person obtaining 262–3
  principle 260
  process 261
  professional responsibilities 261
  records/record keeping 261, 263
  refusal of care by patient 257, 263–4
  types 263
  validity **260**, 261
  verbal 263
  voluntary **260**
  written 263
continuing professional development
      (CPD) 290–4, **295**
  avoiding allegations of negligence 258
  evidence provision 291
  lifelong learning 292
  NMC requirement 291
  Post Registration Education and
      Practice standard 292, 293–4, **295**
  professional portfolio 291, **295**
  starting new job 310–11
control, coping with stress **159**
cost-effectiveness, evidence-based
      practice 180
coursework
  referred 302
  resits 302–3
criminal convictions 7, 25
  data protection 300
  declaring 299

criminal records check 7
  Criminal Records Bureau (CRB) 299–300
  electives 141
critical illness, patients at risk 71
critical thinking skills 215
cross-sectional survey **186**
CUBAN mnemonic 165–6
cultural standards, learned 85
Cumulative Index to Nursing and Allied
    Health Literature (CINAHL)
    183, 187
curriculum
  design 37
  development 35
  flexibility 270
  NMC validation 37
curriculum vitae (CV) 5, **6**
  job applications 307
  professional portfolio 221
  writing **221**

data protection, criminal convictions 300
Data Protection Act (1988), health record
    definition 233
databases 187, **188**, *189*, 190
Databases of Reviews of Effectiveness
    (DARE) 190
death
  practice learning opportunities 303
  reflection 303
decision making 156–7
  capacity 266
  evidence-based practice 182, 185, **187**
  proxy for people lacking capacity 265
  skills 215
degrees 108
delegation
  duty of care 254
  records/record keeping 243
dentists 20
Department of Health
  care record definition 233
  clinical academic careers 276, **277**
  continuing professional
      development 290–4, **295**
  types of records 232, **232–3**
dignity 79
disability adviser 301
Disability Discrimination Act (1995) 301

disclosure of information 87–8
Disclosure Scotland 300
doctors, medical register 20
documentation 230–3
  abbreviations use 241, 242–3
  accuracy 241
  acronym use 242
  all relevant information 237
  clarity 237
  contemporaneous 238
  definition 233
  ELBOW rule **241**
  errors 239, **240**, 241
  facts 237
  good 241
  good nursing care promotion 235
  holistic approach 237
  integrity preservation 239
  legal standards 235–6
  litigation 239
  objective 237, 241
  professional standards 235–6
  reasons for 234–6
  safety maintenance 243–7
  symbols 242
  types 232, **232–3**
  see also records/record keeping
dress style 84
  job interviews 307
drug use, coping with stress 305–6
duty of care 253–5
  breach **255**, **259–60**
  negligence 256, 257, **259–60**
dyslexia 300–1

early warning systems 237
  see also Modified Early Warning Score
      (MEWS)
education 2–3
  careers in 274
  degree-level 35
  funding 3–4
  history 29–30
  NMC role in standards 21–2
  preparation for **11**
  programme 2
  standards 35–7
  starting in 11, **12**, 13
educational development certificates 221

ELBOW rule for documentation **241**
e-learning 111
electives 131–42
  budgeting **137**
  checklist **141**
  contacts 135, **140**
  costs 136–7
  creativity promotion 132
  criminal record screening 141
  duration 132
  funding 132, 136–8, **139**
  getting the most out of it 140–1
  health screens 140–1
  honorary contract 140
  immunisation status 140
  impacts 134
  innovation 132
  location 134
  making contact 139
  malaria protection 141
  memorandum of agreement 140
  nursing process approach **136**
  occupational health clearance 140–1
  organisation 133
  paperwork 135–6
  personal health/safety 141
  planning 139
  preparation 135–6
  processes 135
  programme requirements 133
  protective clothing 141
  purpose 131–4, **135**
  risk assessment 139, **140**
  travel health 141
  uniforms 136
emotions **85**
  reflective cycle 202
employees, duty of care 254
employers
  duty of care 254
  involvement in education
      curriculum 35
entrepreneurship 275
entry to nursing 299–300
environment of care 116–17
essential skills clusters (ESCs) 80–95
  care **81**, 82–3
    organisational aspects 89, **90**
  communication **81**, 82–6, **88**

compassion 80, **81**, 82–3
confidentiality 86–7, 88, **89**
disclosure of information 87–8
infection prevention/control **81**, 90–1
medicines management **81**, 92–3, **94**
numerical assessments 94–5
nutrition and fluid management **81**, 92
organisational aspects of care **81**
everyone counts 80
evidence-based practice 178–88, *189*, 190–2
  accessing evidence 187–8, *189*, 190, **191**
  barriers to implementation 191–2
  care quality 180, **181**, 192
  clinical decisions 185, **187**
  cost-effectiveness 180
  cycle 183–4, **184**
  database searches 187, **188**, *189*, 190
  decision making 182, 185, **187**
  definition 179–81
  eligibility criteria 190
  hierarchies of evidence 185, **185–7**
  levels of evidence **186**
  literature search 187, 188, *189*, 190
  research 180, 181–2, 184, 191
  resources 187–8, *189*, 190, **191**
  sources of evidence 184, **185**
  stages **183**, *184*
exercise, coping with stress **158**, 305
expert opinion **186**
expert patient 46
eyes, nonverbal communication 86

families, involvement 270
feedback 150, **151**
  communication **156**
Fenwick, Ethel Bedford 29
fields of nursing 2, **33**
Fitness to Practice Committees, records 231
fitness to practise 25
five Rs of reflection 204, **205**, **206**
fluid management **81**, 92
freedoms, people without capacity 266
funding arrangements for education 3–4

General Dental Council 20
General Medical Council (GMC) 19–20

General Social Care Council (GSCC)
see Health and Care Professions
Council (HCPC)
Gibbs' reflective cycle 202–4
Glasgow Coma Scale 73–6
components 73
motor response 75
muscle strength assessment 75
neurological status assessment 74–5,
76
pupil size/reaction assessment 76
subjectivity 74
global health 134
good character 7, 25
guidelines 250, 252, **287**
healthcare-associated infection
prevention 90–1
NICE **183**
Scottish Intercollegiate Guidelines
Network **183**

handover of patients
communication 164
computerised sheets 165
confidentiality 165
CUBAN mnemonic 165–6
intentional rounding 163–4, **166**
length 165
location 164, **166**
methods 164–5
structured approach **166**
styles 165
terminology 163–6, **166–7**
time management 166
types 164
verbal 165, **167**
ward handover 164–6
written 165, **167**
handwashing *91*
harm *54*, 55
prevention 56
harmful substances 305–6
health, WHO definition 45
Health and Care Professions Council
(HCPC) 17, **18–19**, 19
professional bodies regulated by **18–19**
registrant duties 19
Health and Social Care Act (2012) 51, **53**
Health and Wellbeing Boards 52

health information, personal 87
health of nurses 25
clearance for university 7, 8
health profession regulation 15–17
health records see records/record keeping
Health Technology Assessment (HTA) 190
healthcare 45–7
costs 43–4, **45**
funding 45
inequalities 45
primary 45–6
provision 43–5
divisions 45–7
reforms 47, **50**, 51–3, 57
requirements 45
secondary 45–6
settings for delivery 35
social care integration 51–2
tax-based funding 45
tertiary 45–6
healthcare records see records/record
keeping
healthcare-associated infections,
guidelines for prevention 90–1
Healthwatch 52, **53**
hearsay 309
high-risk patients, Modified Early
Warning Score 71
holistic approach 147, 237
housing, careers in 274
human rights, confidentiality 87

improving lives 80
independent sector careers 274
infection prevention/control **81**, 90–1
guidelines for healthcare-associated
infections 90–1
information disclosure 87–8
information systems, records/record
keeping 245
in-house training courses 221
integrated care pathway 32
intentional rounding 163–4, **166**
interpersonal skills 22, 153–8, **158–60**
assertiveness 156
communication 155, **155–6**
decision making 156–7
listening skills 154, **154–5**
problem solving 157

professional portfolio 215
   stress management 157–8, **158–60**
interpreters, consent 263
interviews 8–10, **11**
   group 8, 10
   individual 8–10
   job applications 306
   preparation for 9
investigations, duty to assist 308

jargon 167, **168**, **170**
   statement writing 309
job applications
   application form 307
   professional portfolio 306–8
   referees 307
   timing 307
   see also curriculum vitae (CV)
Johari window 148–50, **151–2**
   blind area 150, **151**
   hidden area 150, **151**
   open area 149, **151**
   unknown area 150, **151**
journal clubs 191
journals, peer-reviewed 188

knowledge
   clinical academic careers 278
   generation from reflective
      practice 199, 206
   practice-based 182
   qualified nurses 283
   record in professional portfolio 214,
      215
   research 182
Knowledge and Skills Framework 269
   appraisal process 289
Kolb's learning cycle 201

language use 167–9, **170**
   consent 263
   protocols 251
   statement writing 309
law, common/statute 87
leadership 274–5
learning
   activities 294
   evidence recording 213, **214**
   experiential 123

lifelong 292
non-traditional opportunities 35
outcomes 294
practical 123
process 195
professional portfolio 215, 219, 220,
   224
reflection 195, 199
theoretical 289
verification 224
see also practice learning opportunities
learning cycle 201
learning disability nursing **33**
   practice learning opportunities **119**,
      120
   professional values **40**
legal proceedings
   consent issues 262
   documentation for 235–6
   healthcare record use 234, 235–6
   misconduct 253
legal standards, documentation
      for 235–6
library, university **188**
lifelong learning 292
listening skills 154, **154–5**
literacy 4
literature search 187, 188, *189*, 190
   inclusion/exclusion criteria 190
litigation, documentation/records 239
living wills 264
long-term conditions 46, **46–7**, 269

malaria protection, electives 141
Malnutrition Universal Screening Tool
      (MUST) 66–9, 92
   BMI calculation 67, *68*
   intervention 68, **69**
   risk score 68, **69**
   steps 67
medical register 19, 20
Medicines and Healthcare Products
      Regulatory Agency 15
medicines management **81**, 92–3, **94**
   legal/ethical frameworks 93
MEDLINE **183**, 187
mental capacity 264–5
Mental Capacity Act (2005) 265–6
mental health acts 265–6

mental health nursing **33**
  practice learning opportunities
    119, 120
  professional values **40**
Mental Health (Northern Ireland) Order
    (1986) 265
mentors 124, 125, 128, 282
meta-analysis **185**
Midwives Registration Act (1902) 29
mindmaps 208
minors (under 16 years), consent 264
misconduct
  allegations 253
  negligence 256
mnemonics 165–6, 174, **175**
models of nursing 62, **63**, 64
modern matrons 272
Modified Early Warning Score
    (MEWS) 69–73
  action plan 73
  aims 70
  chart 72
  high-risk patients 71
  physiological measurements 71
  scores triggering action 72–3
  track-and-trigger scoring system 69,
    70, 71, 72
  use 71–2
modules
  failure 302
  re-enrolling 303
  resits 302–3
  retakes 303
Monitor 52
motor response 75
muscle strength assessment 75

National Health Service (NHS)
  employee numbers 44
  services 43–5
National Institute for Health and Care
    Excellence (NICE)
  Glasgow Coma Scale use 74
  guidelines **183**
  track-and-trigger scoring systems 71
National Patient Safety Authority 55
National Union of Students (NUS)
    107
neglect 55

negligence 256–9, **259–60**
  avoiding allegations 258
  breach of duty 256, 257–8
  burden of proof 258
  causation 258
  claims 256
  consent complaints 262
  definition 256
  duty of care 256, 257
    breach **255, 259–60**
  examples 259
  liability 259
  misconduct cases 256
neurological status assessment 74–5, 76
newly registered practitioners 285
  preceptorship 289, **290**
NHS Constitution 79–80, 81
  communication 82
NICE see National Institute for Health and
    Care Excellence (NICE)
night site coordinator 164
Nightingale, Florence 29
Nightingale Training School, St Thomas'
    Hospital (London) 29
numeracy 4
numerical assessments 94–5
nurse consultants 272
nurse–patient relationship 147
Nurses, Midwives and Health Visitors Act
    (1979) 29
Nurses Registration Acts (1919) 29
nursing, definition 28
Nursing and Midwifery Council
    (NMC) 20–1
  behaviour/conduct of students 300
  clinical practice standards 123,
    124, **125**
  code of professional conduct 22–3,
    39, 81
    confidentiality 86–7
    consent issues 262, 263
    duty of care 253
    patient involvement in care 262
    professional portfolio 220
    record keeping 234, **234–5**, 235–6,
    239
    standards 253, 254
  communication 21
  competence standards 283

conduct standards 21–2
consultations 21
continuing professional development
    requirement 291, **295**
curriculum validation 37
degree-level nursing 30, 35
education standards 21–2
essential skills clusters use 80, 81
fitness to practise 25
formation 30
good character 25
guidance on records/record
    keeping 230, 231
health of nurses 25
investigations 22
managing concerns/allegations 22
medicines management standards 93
Post Registration Education and
    Practice standards 291, **291–2**,
    292–4, **295**
    guidance for CPD 294
pre-registration nurse education
    competence 37–9, **40**, 283
    principles for 32–3
    standards for 27–8, 30–41, 178,
    300–1
professional conduct of student
    nurses 23–4
quality assurance 38–9, **40**
register 20, 21, 22
registration with 301–2
regulatory role 20–1
requirements for education 4
Nursing and Midwifery Order (2001) 20
nursing grand rounds 191
nursing process 60, *61*, 62
    elective experience **136**
    phases 60, **61**, 63–4
    steps **63**
nutrition and fluid management
    81, 92
nutritional screening 66–9

obesity 66, **69**
occulesics 86
occupational health clearance for
    electives 140–1
older people, quality of care 83
Open University 100

passwords 245
patient safety 54–5
patients 298
    beliefs 298
    choice provision 270
    documentation of change in
        condition 237
    expert patient 46
    healthcare preferences 46
    information withholding 245
    involvement in care 262
    partner in care 47
    refusal of care 257, 263–4
    standard of care **255**
    values 298
    working together for 80
personal development
    certificates 221
    professional portfolio 215
    reflective practice 207
personal development planning
        (PDP) 105, **106**
    cycle 217–18
    professional portfolio 216–18, 224–5
personal skills 153–8, **158–60**
personal space 85, 86
personal statement, professional
        portfolio 220
personal tutors 104–6, 128
physical activity, coping with stress **158**,
    305
police statement 308
policies 251–2, **253**
    development process *254*
Post Registration Education and Practice
        (PREP) standards 291, **291–2**,
        292–4, **295**
    continuing professional
        development 292, 293–4, **295**
    practice 292, 293, **295**
    record keeping 294
practice learning opportunities 115–25,
        126–7, 128–9
    anxieties 303
    assessment 123–4, **125**
    death 303
    learning 121–3, **125**
    planning 125
    practice placements 117–18

practice learning opportunities *(cont'd)*
  practice setting 115–18
  responsibilities 125, **126–7**, 128
  roles 125, **126–7**, 128
  shared experiences with other
      professions 120–1
  simulation centre 129
  stakeholders 125
  supernumerary practice 128
  teaching 121–3, **125**
practice nurse, handover of patients 164
practice placements 117–18
  planning 125
  responsibilities **126–7**
  supernumerary practice 128
practice-based knowledge 182
preceptors/preceptorship 282, 284–6,
      287, **290**
  continuing professional
    development 290
  core components 289
  definitions 284–5
  elements **288–9**
  framework 287–9, **290**
  guidelines **287**
  implementing 289
  limits 285
  newly registered practitioners 289, **290**
  programmes 287
  records 289
  Scottish programme 287
  starting new job 311
  support for newly qualified health
    professionals 283
  tripartite arrangement 288
pre-registration nurse education 270
  academic level 32
  degree-level 30, 35
  dyslexic students 300–1
  education standards 40–1
  integrated care pathway 32
  length of programme 32
  nature of programme 32
  new standards 34–6
    need for 33–4
  principles 32–3
  professional recognition 32
  professional values 39, **40**
  programme of study 37

quality assurance 38–9, **40**
  standards 27–8, 30–41, 178, 300–1
    for competence 37–9, **40**, 283
    education 40–1
pressure ulcers, assessment tool 65–6
preventive medicine 269
primary care 269
Primary Care Trusts, abolition 52, **53**
problem solving skills 157
  professional portfolio 215
  reflection 199
procedures 250
PRODIGY **183**
professional accountability 283
professional bodies *56*, 57
professional conduct
  NMC code 22–3
  student nurses 23–4, 300
  see also misconduct
professional development
  reflective practice 207
  see also continuing professional
    development (CPD)
professional portfolio 212–28
  action plans 224–5
  assessments from others 223
  competence documentation 212, 215
  compilation **224**
  components 213, **214**
  confidentiality 212–13, 223
  content 218–25, **225–6**
  continuing professional
    development 291, **295**
  critical thinking skills 215
  curriculum vitae 221
  decision-making skills 215
  educational development
    certificates 221
  e-portfolio (digital) 226–7
  evidence of growth/achievement 213,
    214–15
  format 226–7
  in-house training courses 221
  interpersonal skills 215
  introduction 220
  job applications 306–8
  knowledge record 214, 215
  learning outcomes 215, 219, 220
  learning verification 224

need for 214–18
paper portfolio 226
personal aims, objectives,
    aspirations 213
personal development certificates 221
personal development planning
    216–18, 224–5
personal growth 215
personal statement 220
problem solving skills 215
reflection 215
reflection/reflective practice **214**
representative 225
selective 225
self-analysis/feedback 222
skills record 214
staff nurse post application 306–8
structure 218–25, **225–6**
table of contents 220
work history 221
professional standards, documentation
    for 235–6
Professional Standards Authority for
    Health and Social Care (PSA) 15–17
Project 2000 29–30
protective clothing 141
protocols 249–51, **253**
    abbreviations use 251
    accountability 251
    advantages 250, **251**
    definition 249
    details associated with **250**
    disadvantages 250, **251**
    language use 251
    parts 250
psychomotor skills 21
Public Concern at Work *56*, 57
public health **53**, 269
    reforms 52
Public Health England 52
public interest 88
pupil size/reaction assessment 76

qualified nurses *see* registered nurses
qualities of nurses 21
Quality Assurance Agency for Higher
    Education (QAA) 98, 99
    personal development planning
        216–17

quality of care
    commitment to 79
    evidence-based practice 180, **181**, 192
    older people 83

randomised controlled trial (RCT) **186**
reasonable care standard 254
reasoning, five Rs of reflection 204, **205**
reconstructing, five Rs of reflection 204,
    205
records/record keeping 230–9, **240**, 241–7
    abbreviations use 241, 242–3
    access 244–5
    accuracy 241
    acronym use 242
    archiving 245
    closure 245
    communication facilitation 235
    complaints investigation 231
    confidentiality 244
    consent 261, 263
    contemporaneous 238
    definition 233
    delegation 243
    documentation 230–3
        legal/professional standards 235–6
        reasons for 234–6
    ELBOW rule **241**
    errors 239, **240**, 241
    function 234
    good nursing care promotion 235
    guidance for keeping **234–5**
    information systems 245
    integrity preservation 239
    legal proceedings use 234, 235–6
    litigation 239
    minimum retention period 246
    NMC code of professional conduct 234,
        234–5, 235–6, 239
    objective 237, 241
    Post Registration Education and
        Practice standards 294
    preceptorship 289
    principles 237–9, **240**, 241
    safe disposal 245–7
    safety maintenance 243–7
    security 245
    symbols 242
    time for holding 245–6

referees 307
reflection 147
  on action/in action 200–1
  death 303
  definition 195–7
  guided on practice 289
  learning process 195, 199
  personal qualities 197, **197–8**
  problem solving skills 199
  process 199
  professional portfolio **214**, 215
  self-awareness 199, 206
  strengths 198, 207
  value 206–9
reflective cycle 202–4
reflective practice 195–204, **205**, 206–10
  awareness of thoughts/feelings 199
  bridge between theory and
      practice 199
  definition 196, 197
  frameworks 200–1, 204, **205, 206**
  Gibbs' reflective cycle 202–4
  knowledge generation 199, 206
  Kolb's learning cycle 201
  models 200–4
  personal development 207
  practical issues 206–7
  professional development 207
  professional portfolio **214**
  supervision 289
  value 206–9
  writing 207–8
registered nurses
  competence 256, 283
  expectations 283
  professional accountability 283
  transition from student 282, 283, 284
Regulation and Quality Improvement
    Agency (Northern Ireland) 15
relating, five Rs of reflection 204, **205**
relaxation techniques **158**, 306
reporting, five Rs of reflection 204, **205**
research
  evidence-based practice 180, 181–2,
      184, 191
  knowledge 182
  process 182
  skills development 275
  see also clinical academic careers

respect 79
responding, five Rs of reflection 204, **205**
rest, coping with stress **159**
rights
  human rights in confidentiality 87
  people without capacity 266
Royal College of Nursing (RCN) 107
  definition of nursing 28

safeguarding of adults
  advocate role 56
  concerns, raising and escalating *56*, 57
  guidance 56–7
  people lacking capacity 264–5
  principles 54
  speaking out 55–7
  support 56–7
safety briefing 165–6
saying 'no,' coping with stress
      159, 160
schools, careers in 274
Schools of Nursing 99
Scottish Intercollegiate Guidelines
    Network (SIGN) **183**
security, records/record keeping 245
self-analysis/feedback, professional
      portfolio 222
self-awareness 147–50, **151–2**
  feedback 150, **151**
  Johari window 148–50, **151–2**
  reflection 199, 206
self-care 269
self-help 47
self-management 143–50, **151–2**, 153–8,
      158–9
  assertiveness 156, **159**
  assumptions 145
  attitudes 145
  beliefs 144–5, **146–7**
  communication skills 155, **155–6**
  decision making 156–7
  health 270
  interpersonal skills 153–8, **158–60**
  listening skills 154, **154–5**
  personal skills 153–8, **158–60**
  problem solving skills 157
  self-awareness 147–50, **151–2**
    Johari window 148–50, **151–2**
  self-reflection 147

stress management 157–8, **158–60**, 304–6
    values 144–5, **146–7**
self-medication 47
self-reflection 147
service providers 128
service provision 34–6
SIGN (Scottish Intercollegiate Guidelines Network) **183**
simulation centre 129
skills of nurses 21–2, 283
    clinical academic careers 278
    clusters 283
    communication skills 155, **155–6**
    listening skills 154, **154–5**
    record in professional portfolio 214
    see also interpersonal skills; problem solving skills
sleep, coping with stress **158–9**
smartcards 245
smoking 305–6
social care 47–50
    challenges 49–50
    costs 43–4, **45**
    healthcare integration 51–2
    partnership working 49, 50
    principles 49
    provision 43–5
    reform requirements 45
    reforms 47, **50**, 51–3, 57
    staff 48
    user numbers 48
social exclusion 45
social inclusion 49
social services, careers in 274
social work 49
social work assistants 48
social workers 48–9
staff nurse post application 306–8
statement writing 308–10
    format 309–10
    preparation 308–9
Strategic Health Authorities, abolition 52, **53**
stress management 157–8, **158–60**, 304–6
    coping strategies 305–6
student nurses
    bullying 304
    competence 283
    conduct 300
    duty of care 255
    dyslexia 300–1
    expectations 282
    failing assignments 302–3
    inappropriate behaviour 300
    professional conduct 23–4
    stress management 304–6
    transition to qualified nurse 282, 283, 284
student representative bodies 107, **108**
student support services 103–6
supernumerary practice 128
SWOT analysis **222–3**
symbols, documentation/records 242
systematic review **185**

talking, coping with stress 306
teaching, practice learning opportunities 121–3
teamwork 19
terminology 162–76
    abbreviations 168–9
    acronym use 169
    anatomical landmarks 170–2
    communication **170**
    jargon 167, **168**, **170**
    language 167–9, **170**
    mnemonics 165–6, 174, **175**
    nursing handover 163–6, **166–7**
    prefixes/suffixes 172–3, **173–4**
therapeutic relationship 147
time management
    coping with stress **159**
    handover of patients 166
tobacco use 305–6
track-and-trigger scoring system 69, 70, 71, 72
trade unions *56*, 57
training courses, in-house 221
transferrable skills 269–70
travel health for electives 141
treatment, documentation of omissions 237

UK Central Council for Nursing Midwifery and Health Visiting (UKCC) 29, 30
UK Clinical Research Collaboration 278
UK Medical Act (1983) 20

undergraduate nursing programme
  content 98
  see also curriculum
undernutrition 66
uniforms 84
  electives 136
UNISON 107
universities 2, 98–114
  academic staff 101, **101–2**
  academic year 108–9
  advice and guidance session 302
  application 4–5
  application form 5, **6**
  assessment 110–13
  blended learning 111
  bullying management 304
  categories **99**
  choice 2–3
  criminal records check 7, 25
  declaring criminal convictions 299
  degree classification **108**
  entry requirements 4–5
  failing assignments 302–3
  fitness to practise 25
  health clearance 7, 8, 25
  institution 99
  interviews 7–8, 8–10, **11**
  learning 110–13
  libraries **188**
  modular credits 109–10
  offer of a place 10
  personal statement 5, **6**
  personal tutors 104–6
  preparation for starting **11**
  professional administrative staff 102
  programme of study 108–13, 111
  research 100
  selection days 7–8
  senior management team 100
  structure 100–2, **103**
  student representative bodies 107, **108**
  student support services 103–6
  support staff 102
  teaching 100, 110–13
  Vice Chancellor 100

values
  patient 298
  personal of nurses 144–5, **146–7**
Vice Chancellor 100
voluntary sector careers 274
vulnerable adults 53–5, 56
  definition 53

ward handover 164–6
Waterlow pressure ulcer assessment
    tool 65–6
well-being promotion 147
whistleblowing *55*
witness statement 308
word roots 172, **173**
work history, professional portfolio 221
work opportunities 1–2
workforce requirements 271–2
Working in Partnership Programme
    (2006), protocol definition 249
workplace, learning in 122–3
World Health Organization (WHO),
    health definition 45
writing, reflective 207–8